Nursing Children

Nursing Children

Psychology, research and practice

Third edition

Jayne Taylor BSc (Hons) Nursing, RGN, RHV, Dip. N (Lond), Cert Ed
Director of Nursing and Midwifery, Suffolk College
Ipswich, Suffolk, UK

Dave Müller BEd, PhD, C.Psychol FBPsS
Vice Principal, Suffolk College
Ipswich, Suffolk, UK

Lesley Wattley BA (Hons), RGN
Formerly Senior Lecturer, North East Surrey College of Technology
Surrey, UK

Pam Harris BSc, MA, PhD, ABPsS, C.Psychol
Faculty of Community Health Sciences
University of Wales Institute, Cardiff, Wales

Stanley Thornes (Publishers) Ltd

First edition published by Harper & Row, 1986
Second edition published 1992
Third edition published in 1999 by
Stanley Thornes (Publishers) Ltd
Ellenborough House
Wellington Street
Cheltenham
GL50 1YW
UK

A catalogue record for this book is available from the British Library.

ISBN 0 7487 3327 2

99 00 01 02 03 / 10 9 8 7 6 5 4 3 2 1

Typeset by Acorn Bookwork, Salisbury, Wilts
Printed and bound in Great Britain by Martins The Printers Ltd., Berwick upon Tweed

CONTENTS

ACKNOWLEDGEMENTS

The authors wish to thank a number of individuals for their practical help and general encouragement during the writing of this book. These include Action for Sick Children, Barbara Weller, John Harris, Vik Müller and Stewart Taylor. Special thanks to Neil Bray for his photographic contributions.

ACKNOWLEDGEMENTS

PREFACE

This new and revised version of this book maintains the unashamedly psychological emphasis of previous editions. We have not rejected the physical aspects of medicine, nor have we questioned the need for the provision of medical care by qualified personnel. We do, however, demonstrate that physical care is linked inextricably to the psychological wellbeing of children.

In this up to date version of the book we have been able to put together even more evidence to show the importance of providing psychological as well as physical support, both of which contribute towards the holistic care of children and their families. Even 13 years on from the publication of the original version there is still not enough emphasis given to the psychological aspects of the care of children, especially during initial nurse education. Hopefully, this will gradually change. This book has been updated to help facilitate this change and to encourage nurses at all levels to draw upon research findings in their work with children.

Nurses no longer seem put off as much as they have in the past by the notion of psychology and it is now well established that nursing is a research based profession. The links between psychology and research are inextricable and it remains clear to us that a great deal of nursing research shows similar methods and approaches to the study of psychology.

What has always been important about undertaking research into nursing is that it should be of practical value. We believe that the research included in this book, especially that undertaken more recently, has enormous implications for nursing practice and indeed is guiding a great deal of current thinking within the field. At the end of each chapter we have drawn out in an almost prescriptive manner how we think the body of research reported should affect practice. We do not apologise for this and believe that it is important to tease out the practical implications of the knowledge which we have gained through research and practice over the last decade.

The original version of the book was produced by Dave Müller, Pam Harris and Lesley Wattley. The major responsibility for revising it and bringing it up to date for the second, and for this edition has fallen to Jayne Taylor. Dave Müller worked closely with Jayne and in particular drew upon his experience as an applied psychologist and writer in supporting the revision. We would both wish to pay enormous tribute to the work undertaken by Lesley Wattley and Pam Harris in producing what was then an innovative text in the field of the psychology of nursing children.

The first part of the book was originally produced by Lesley Wattley and Pam Harris to convey to the reader some of the excitement of studying child development which we believe has been retained. Throughout the chapters the relevance of research is stressed and set firmly in a nursing context. Indeed, the chapters were selected to be of relevance to the practice of nursing and therefore as a review of child psychology the part is not comprehensive; but as a collection of key topics in the field for nurses we think that it still achieves our aims.

The second part of the book depended heavily on the knowledge that Pam Harris gained from her own research into this topic. We have been able to update this part and to add two chapters, including an additional chapter on community child care which we feel takes Pam's original work a stage further. We believe that this very important topic should be included in the light of recent developments. As a part it can still be read independently of the rest of the book and we hope it will be useful not only to nurses, but to parents as well. It would be interesting to hear from any of our readers, especially parents, about their views on any of the issues we have raised.

The third part is more specialized and includes a range of the problems and challenges that nurses face. Of those selected we do feel that the topics cover the major issues facing nurses working and caring for children and we hope that you find them of practical value. This part now includes an important chapter on HIV for which Jayne took major responsibility. All the other areas have also been updated and, in particular, the chapter on child abuse has, as in the second edition, been significantly rewritten to bring it more in line with current thinking. Despite the two of us taking front line responsibility for producing this book we have kept true to the spirit of the original version and have consulted both Pam and Lesley in producing it.

Our final chapter, although an overview, is still more of a policy statement. Here we draw together a number of factors which we feel should be taken into account in nursing children. We hope we have provided enough evidence in this chapter to continue to influence people and for you, the reader, to become responsible for improving the nursing care given to children and adolescents, both physiologically and psychologically. We hope you enjoy this book.

Jayne Taylor and Dave Müller
in collaboration with Pam Harris and Lesley Wattley

PART ONE

THE DEVELOPING CHILD

Psychology, Children and Nursing

1

Infants and children are sometimes so desperately ill that all clinical efforts must be urgently directed at trying to ensure their physical survival. For the majority of children though, illness and injury are not sudden, dramatic, life threatening events and there is normally an opportunity for nurses to consider not just the children's medical problems but also their emotional, social and developmental needs. However, it is uncertain whether these needs are always being met or even fully considered (Thomas, 1994; House of Commons, 1997a). For example, few paediatric nursing text books address psychological issues in any depth, concentrating instead on the physical aspects of illness and on the skills concerned with medical care and treatment. Similarly, the education of nurses and midwives has, in the past, tended to emphasize physical rather than psychological knowledge.

This problem has not however gone unrecognized. An active pressure group, Action for Sick Children, is continuing to campaign to enlighten hospitals about aspects of practical management on issues such as parental participation in care at all times and the development of facilities and free accommodation for parents on children's wards. It also serves to disseminate research findings as does The National Children's Bureau which documents research and supplies abstracts and bibliographies concerning the care of children. In addition, official reports have been produced which clearly state policies concerning the psychosocial and emotional needs of children in hospital and the community. These include the Platt report (1959), the Court report (1976), and the more recent reports The Welfare of Children and Young People in Hospital (Department of Health 1991), Children First (Audit Commission, 1993), Child Health in the Community (Department of Health, 1996), The Specific Health Needs of Children and Young People (House of Commons, 1997b) and Health Services for Children and Young People: Home and School (House of Commons, 1997a). Finally, the Children Act (Department of Health, 1989), which made major changes in child law, has particular implications for children with special needs and children who have been abused.

Many of the recommended changes made in recent reports are within the scope of nurses, and could be made without major additional staffing or finance. Historically, however, those involved in child care services have a poor record of acting upon such reports. This was shown by reports undertaken by the Consumers' Association (1980, 1985), which surveyed practices in hospitals in relation to the specific recommendations of the Platt report (1959). It was found that, although great improvements had been made, children in some hospitals were still

Action for Sick Children (previously NAWCH), 300 Kingston Road, Wimbledon Chase, London SW20 8LX
Tel: 0181-542 4848
Fax: 0181-542 2424
National Children's Bureau, 8 Wakley Street, Islington, London EC1V 7QE. Tel: 0171-278 9441

experiencing restriction of parental presence in the hospital; outmoded attitudes towards other visitors, especially siblings; the continued practice of treating children on adult wards, which is considered harmful; absence of pre-admission visits; inadequate information leaflets; mixed adult/child outpatient facilities; low priority on the part of some ward sisters regarding individual patient assignment.

The 1980 report stated that 'it emerged that generally the most powerful factor determining the way the children were treated was the attitude of the hospital staff'. This finding is both pessimistic and optimistic. On the one hand, it is sad that the attitudes of hospital staff have led to such an unsatisfactory state of affairs. On the other hand, there does exist the possibility of helping people modify their attitudes and to make them more sympathetic to the knowledge that is currently available concerning children. Furthermore, this may not require vast sums of money to implement, unlike shortages of staff or inadequate buildings.

ASSUMPTIONS IN CHILD CARE

As with nursing traditions, cultural beliefs about childrearing practices are rarely based on the results of carefully conducted research. Similarly, beliefs about the 'right way' to raise children are just as susceptible to the prevailing moral attitudes of a culture as some nursing practices are to fashions and the traditions of particular hospitals, though we may not recognize this at the time. We bring to our actions certain views about how things should be done, but often they are little more than opinions or habits. A good example of a change in opinions is toilet training. Thirty years ago it was thought this was best achieved by the time the child was 1 year old, but now it is regarded in a much more relaxed manner. Similarly, we may believe that children are intrinsically 'good' or naturally 'bad'. In the last century there were several schools of thought on this issue which may have influenced childrearing practices. An extreme view was that children were born 'evil' and could only be 'saved' if their naturally selfish wills were broken through absolute obedience to adult demands. On the other hand, a more romantic view was that children were essentially 'good' and a parent's task was to preserve this state. These ideas have been described by Sunley (1955, p. 151) who illustrates the role of the more tender parent with this quotation from *Letters to Young Mothers* written in 1838 by a woman called Lydia Sigourney.

> *Nurture the infant ... as a germ quickened by spring ...*
> *opens the folding doors of its little heart ... like*
> *timid tendrils seeking where to twine.*

Romantic beliefs such as these may affect people's reactions to children, for example in deciding whether to cuddle or ignore a crying baby, or to encourage or discourage playfulness.

Although these particular ideas may seem curious today, it is important to recognize the factors which may have played a subtle role in shaping and influencing our thinking. If we can stand back a little from our opinions and beliefs and try to test or investigate them, we may find more substantial reasons for carrying out care in particular ways. In the next section we will examine in more detail some of the important assumptions underlying current attitudes towards childrearing which psychologists have been investigating.

THE EFFECTS OF CHILDHOOD EXPERIENCE

Why do we bring up our children in certain predictable ways? Why is it we have books full of instructions for new parents on how to raise children successfully? Why are we so very self-conscious in our approaches to child care? What are the consequences we fear if we were to get it wrong? These are examples of common questions parents and others are likely to think about at some time. People have long been fascinated by what makes one person a diplomat and another a spy; one an upright citizen and another a criminal. If we knew the answer to this, so the argument goes, we could cure the world of its 'diseases' of violence, aggression and greed. This is an attractive idea, based on the belief that the way children are brought up will have permanent effects on their physical health, their mental state, their ability to make social relationships, the kind of society they create, and even the world they live in. Many writers have stated this sort of belief from the time of Plato to the present day. Kagan *et al.* (1978) discuss some of them in their very interesting book on infancy, where they quote the following, written in 1796.

> *Were man able to trace every effect to its cause he would probably find that the virtue or vice of an individual, the happiness or misery of a family, the glory or infamy of a nation, have had their sources in the cradle over which the prejudices of a nurse or mother have presided. The years of infancy are those in which the chains of virtue or vice are generally forged.*

This quotation illustrates another fundamental assumption about child-rearing: that we can control it, or rather that 'mother figures' can. (This second assumption is discussed on p. 7.)

The ability to love is an important theme running through the literature on child care. In the 1950s, Bowlby made bold claims regarding the nature and quality of mother–infant relationships (Bowlby, 1951). A key theme in his writings was that early caring relationships made it possible for individuals to love in later life. He described 'affectionless characters' who had been deprived of the opportunity to love and for whom this would be a permanent disability. Bowlby drew his evidence from a variety of sources, among which were some studies carried out in foreign orphanages in the 1940s where it was noted that young children under certain circumstances failed to develop appropriately, either physically or psychologically. Bowlby concluded that infants need to have a close, intimate relationship with one caregiver, usually the mother.

Evidence such as this reinforced the commonsense view that the way one is brought up has serious implications both for the individual and for society. For example, as a result of Bowlby's influential work, a World Health Organization Expert Committee (1951) declared that permanent damage would be caused to the emotional health of a future generation if day nurseries and crèches were encouraged as an acceptable form of child care arrangement. Bowlby's (1951) work continues to be influential, but should this be so?

Criticism of Bowlby's work has accumulated gradually as the enormous amount of research his ideas inspired has been published. Clarke and Clarke (1976), who examined the evidence for the significance of early experience, point out that – in the studies from which Bowlby drew his conclusions – conditions in some of the institutions were such that it was not simply maternal care that was missing, but also essential elements of general and physical care. Furthermore, it is surprisingly difficult to substantiate claims that the problems of an individual, a society or of a nation, have their roots in the early experience of infants. A study by Douglas (1975) tried to assess whether disturbed adolescents had been damaged emotionally as a result of childhood admissions to hospital. He found that though a single admission was not associated with an increased risk of delinquency, repeated or prolonged hospital admissions might have been a factor. This work has been criticized by Rutter (1975), who found in his own study that repeated hospital admissions were associated with later disturbance if the first admissions occurred before the age of 5 years. However, there was an important added factor in this study which indicated that children with multiple admissions also often come from disadvantaged homes. This may be an example of the subtle relationship between children's environment and their development. Perhaps similar factors were exerting effects in the studies Bowlby used, although these were not made explicit as they are in Rutter's study.

Here, then, we begin to see an important trend in the thinking of psychologists with regard to the effects of early experience on later life: it is often not a single traumatic event which leads to problems, but several problems or enduring problems which, with their cumulative effects, wear down the individual's resilience. As we shall see in Chapter 2, this is an important point because, for example, the theories of 'bonding' have in the past predicted problems for parents and children if single opportunities for intimate interaction are not exploited in a short, sensitive period after birth. A belief such as this, if carelessly communicated to parents, could become a self-fulfilling prophecy by causing parents to focus on a single 'failure' which may have been unavoidable. This point is also relevant to children's experience of hospitalization, which is discussed further in Chapter 7. If a single event does have long lasting effects of a damaging kind, then the picture is very pessimistic indeed, and parents would be more likely to feel failures from day one. Fortunately, however, current research does tend to suggest that this is not so and that there is no single psychological event which can fully determine a child's future experience of life.

DOES MOTHER KNOW BEST?

Another strongly held assumption in our society is that we can control early development, and that it is the mother who is usually the best person to do this. This assumption is so closely linked to the one concerning the lasting effects of early experience, that it is almost indistinguishable from it. The following quotation, reputed to be a Chinese proverb, comes from the Sunday Express Baby Book (p. 50) available in the 1950s, edited by Woodman:

> *Mother, you have the greatest power in your hands, for where there is harmony in the home, there is peace in the world.*

The enormous implications of statements such as these which, as Rutter (1975) reminds us, have mostly been made by men, have not been lost on women sympathetic to feminism in its various forms: 'Men rule the world and women get the blame because they raised them.' However we cannot be too dismissive of the apparently commonsense view of the mother as the primary caregiver. We must continue the search for an objective basis for our views.

Bowlby, and many other writers, placed so much stress on the importance of the mother for the child's psychological development that the father has apparently been viewed as redundant and unnecessary. Commonsense suggests that this is an unreasonable viewpoint, but it is only comparatively recently that research has turned seriously to assessing the quality of relationships an infant might have with others. It was never really clear to what extent the mother was expected to have continuous or exclusive contact with her infant, or up until what age she was expected to stay with her child, or whether the absence of others, despite her presence, could affect an infant for good or ill. The exclusiveness of the mother's role raised several important questions, not least concerning survival.

One way of looking at any behaviour is to see how much it contributes to the likelihood of survival. Infants, who can respond and become attached to a number of people, presumably enhance their chances of survival. Wolkind and Rutter (1985) suggest that infants are capable of multiple attachments, and these are not exclusively dependent on the amount of time each person spends with the infant, or whether or not they provide care and food. It would appear that it is the quality of interaction, even over a short period of time, which seems to be a particularly salient feature. The absence of the mother for various periods may be no more associated with infant distress or disrupted attachment than, for example, the absence of the father who happens to go out to work every day. Other factors such as the quality of the home environment and other caregivers are also extremely important (Deater-Deckard *et al.*, 1996). Schaffer (1990) found a variety of other people who were important to the infant, such as neighbours, siblings and grandparents, but the persons for whom the infants often had particular attachments were their fathers. Schaffer concludes that usually the belief that a mother is the right person to give care is derived mostly from the fact that she typically does it, than from any more important factor. In other words it results from a cultural rather than a biological influence.

Another limitation of the assumption that mothers are more vital than fathers, is revealed by research into their influence on the development of sex role behaviour. From Lamb's (1981) review of research in this field it appears that mothers and fathers play different roles which enhance the behaviour of boys and girls in different ways. Fathers tend to play more with their children, while mothers often give most of the care. When mothers do play, it is likely to be less physical than that of the father. Mothers tend to discourage exploration, while fathers encourage their babies' curiosity. Lamb (1981, p. 25) concludes from a mass of research literature that one of the best established findings concerning the father is:

> *The masculinity of sons and femininity of daughters is greatest when fathers are nurturant and participate extensively in childrearing. Therefore the father's similarity to a caricatured stereotype of masculinity is far less influential than his involvement in what are often portrayed as female activities.*

In addition to evidence relating to the father's role in sex role behaviour, there is some evidence of his significance in the intellectual and moral development of offspring. Lamb proposes that fathers play an extremely important role in child development.

SOME CRITICISMS

Interestingly, in the studies investigating the father's role, some important limitations in the way the research has been conducted have been noted. For example, what the father does has often been investigated indirectly by asking the children or the mother, which is clearly not satisfactory (Lamb, 1981) as there is no guarantee that either of these sources will provide accurate information or a complete picture. This demonstrates the need of those wanting to implement research findings to be able to evaluate research and recognize any limitations in methodology or interpretation. Another interesting criticism of work in the general field of early relationships is that it has often concentrated exclusively on the reactions of the child. For instance, it seems that children between the ages of 6 months and 6 years who have been separated from the primary caregiver often react to this experience in a particular way. Robertson and Robertson (1989), who studied the separation responses of children for over 30 years, describe how, at first, the child shows signs of protest and cries, refusing any attempt by others to get close and give care. There is then a period labelled 'despair', when the child is quiet and shows very little interest in anything. Finally, there is a period called 'detachment', when the child appears to accept the situation and this has often been thought to mean that the child has settled and is being good ('quiet children are good children'). This kind of research focusses on the child and looks at the disruption of behaviour and relationships in terms of the child. It might also imply that once the child is able to go home from hospital, everything will return to normal. However, as Robertson and Robertson (1989) point out, this is not always the case. Sometimes there are quite severe problems after discharge. One possible reason for this, which Schaffer (1977) has proposed and which appears not to have received much study in humans, is the effect of the separation on primary caregivers and their ability to interpret the signals from their children which normally enable smooth interaction. Schaffer describes the work of Hinde in this context, who demonstrated that the disturbances of the behaviour in an infant monkey following separation from the mother were due primarily to changes in the mother's behaviour as a result of the separation. Naturally, there are always problems in using animal studies to illustrate human phenomena, but perhaps they help us keep our minds open to consider human possibilities.

RESEARCH IN CHILD DEVELOPMENT

One of the unsettling things about research, especially for the person who is unfamiliar with it, is that new results frequently call into question the findings of previous work. A good example is the work on the effects of separation on the child when in hospital. Bowlby's (1951) work was very influential in indicating the great distress that separation could cause. However, as time passes practices and ideas change and a review of relevant research by Schaffer (1990) found the evidence unconvincing and concluded that separation 'is never a "pure" experience that has only the one ingredient i.e. the mother's absence'. Schaffer goes on to provide a detailed and interesting discussion of the other possible influences affecting the nature of stress experienced by some children in hospital, drawing on research into their social experience prior to hospitalization. Thus, hospitalization itself (and separation *per se*) appear not to be the sole factors in causing distress, as Bowlby's work may have suggested.

This freedom to criticize is part of the process of subjecting theories or 'hunches' to rigorous testing to try to establish what is or is not accurate. Although it is difficult, the researcher must be objective and try to ensure that subjective opinions and beliefs are not biasing the findings. As already mentioned, we are susceptible to the assumptions of our society, but one way of trying to ensure that such influences are minimized is to think of ways of investigating human behaviour and experience which can be measured and compared, perhaps with other societies or cultures. Research findings often generate more research ideas so that someone else may look at the same problem in a different way. For example, Rutter (1975) criticized a study by Douglas (1975) on early experience and delinquency and then went on to look at this area himself. He examined fresh data but took into account some other factors which it was thought might better explain the results of Douglas's study (see p. 6, above). Rutter's study identified the presence of an extra factor to explain Douglas's results: that is that a poor home background affected the delinquency rate of children with multiple hospital admissions. Thus, we gradually acquire a clearer picture of the principles of child development by rigorous testing and questioning of the conclusions which emerge.

Methods of research

Many methods of psychological research used in studying children may already be familiar, especially questionnaires, interviews, and rating scales. Psychologists also carry out experiments, undertake observation and may use experiential techniques such as role play (Wattley and Müller, 1984). With children these methods sometimes have to be modified. For example, a very young child may not understand a rating scale that requires numerical answers such as that shown below:

	Not at all	A bit	Very much
How much do you like fish?	1	2	3

They may however happily use a pictorial scale of smiley faces and find it more entertaining (Figure 1.1)

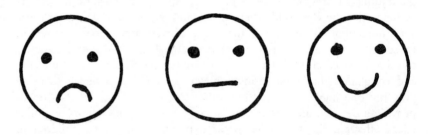

Figure 1.1

Smiley faces rating scale.

Similarly a child may not be able to role-play to order, despite being able to play mums and dads in the play house at school.

Instead, one method which has been used to infer children's understanding of roles, expressions of preference, or emotions, is simply to put them in a room containing various toys and see which ones they play with and how they construct their play. A simple example would be to place dolls, cars, cookery equipment and other toys which might be associated with the play of either boys or girls, and see if the children show any particular preferences, but without priming them as to the nature of the activity. This is also a technique which can be used to investigate the nature of problems of troubled children, and can be used as a way of helping them express themselves. This is often referred to as 'play therapy' and is clearly demonstrated in Axline's (1964) book *Dibs in Search of Self*.

Use of experiments

Experiments have been carried out in many areas of child development. Here the researcher manipulates one or more features of the environment under controlled conditions and measures and records patterns of reactions or behaviour under those conditions. Sometimes, but not always, these experiments call for sophisticated equipment but, in many cases, ingenuity is the order of the day. For example, in one early experiment designed to assess babies' ability to discriminate between faces, a domestic colander was used to simulate facial features (Carpenter, 1974). A certain lack of self-consciousness and a sense of humour is also helpful when, as in one early experiment, a person is required to pop up repeatedly from beneath a table to attract the baby's attention and reward certain behaviour (Bower, 1966).

Observation techniques

Observation is perhaps the most important form of investigation in child psychology and one particular observation technique, developed from ethology, has been especially influential. Ethology has two important concerns: the context in which behaviour occurs, and the adaptive value of that behaviour. Adaptation refers to the biological capacity of an organism or species to respond to its environment in such a way as to ensure its own continued existence. There has been much debate as to whether certain behaviours are inborn, or learnt (sometimes referred to as the nature–nurture debate), and psychologists have observed human beings to see whether they can identify particular behaviours which could be said to support either view. For this reason, observation was carried out in natural settings because it was assumed that an animal (or human) was adapted to that particular setting, and that therefore any behaviour was likely to be specifically relevant to that context. Of course there are still problems such as intrusiveness of the observer, especially if a camera or other equipment is used. However, it is from this approach to the study of people and animals that we derive the survival argument for the potential significance of, for example, multiple attachments in infancy.

Sometimes cross-cultural observation studies are particularly useful in helping to identify the assumptions which influence the childrearing patterns in our society. One example would be Levy-Shiff's (1983) observations of children brought up in the community of the kibbutz in Israel. Among other things, he was able to show that children could develop appropriately, even if not in the continuous presence of the mother, and that they also developed strong relationships with their natural mothers. Another observation was made among South American Indians called the Yequana, who apparently entrust most childminding activities to very young siblings. As Leidloff (1978, pp. 77–8) reported:

I saw little Yequana girls from the age of 3 or 4 taking full charge of infants ... When she is old enough to consider alternative methods, she is already a longstanding expert in baby care.

Throughout this book we will refer to various pieces of research which have been used to understand child development, and it will be helpful to reflect on whether the studies were carried out objectively, systematically and in such a way that they could be replicated. We need to develop skills in the critical analysis of findings before we implement them into practice.

THE NURSING PERSPECTIVE

Throughout this chapter we have made reference to the fact that children and their families, as well as researchers and nurses, are products of and are influenced by the context in which they live. Nurses are in daily contact with parents from a variety of different social backgrounds and cultures, and they hold various values reflecting their own educational, religious and social perspectives. Parents will often turn very willingly to 'experts' such as doctors and nurses for advice, and expect them to be well informed on those matters which affect their children. Many nurses (especially students) care for sick children, never having been parents themselves and certainly without the practice of the little Yequana children to whom traditional childrearing wisdom is passed on at an early age. In the absence of the opportunity to absorb such traditional knowledge, it is perhaps not surprising that we turn to books and pamphlets, but it is vital that, as professional caregivers, we ensure that we recognize the status of the knowledge we use. Otherwise we may simply impose on others opinions and beliefs derived solely from untested assumptions.

Few nurses would deny that physical and psychological wellbeing are intimately linked. However, unless we have a thorough awareness of the psychological as well as the physical needs of children, it is hard to see how this can be taken into account when planning and giving care, nor by what criteria the care may be evaluated. Findings from psychology will not tell us how to nurse children, but they can give us pointers and broaden our understanding of the child's needs, even though we cannot have the experience of researching each issue ourselves.

In practice ➤

- Nurses need to develop awareness of their own opinions and beliefs about the way children should be raised, and to ask themselves if they have any right to impose these onto the children in their care.
- Similarly, nurses need to develop understanding and to be aware of the opinions and beliefs of others, such as parents, children, doctors, etc.

- It is important to be able to recognize where nursing practices are not based on any scientific rationales, and to search for such knowledge. Nurses should be aiming to foster 'research-mindedness' in relation to nursing children.
- It can be very helpful to try and identify the 'survival value' of behaviours of children and families when faced with an unfamiliar situation such as outpatients or a hospital ward. Quietness, for example, may not always be a sign that everything is fine.
- It is sensible to bear in mind that single events, such as brief separation, are not necessarily causal factors in long term distress. Rather, that the cumulative effects of experiences, including those which occur outside hospital in the home (e.g. impoverished or hostile relationships, apathetic parents), can have serious developmental effects.
- As children are not brought up in isolation, we need to try and see them in relation to others. For example, we should try to appreciate the effect of the child on parents, siblings, grandparents and friends, as well as the effects that these people have on the child.
- Nurses, health visitors and midwives should reflect on the variety of roles they play in caring for children and their families. Consideration needs to be given to the extent to which nurses of children are particularly vulnerable to becoming over-involved emotionally, and whether there is a need for special support for nurses as their traditional role in the care of children changes.

REFERENCES

Audit Commission (1993) *Children First*, Audit Commission, London.

Axline, V. (1964) *Dibs in Search of Self*, Penguin, Harmondsworth.

Bower, T.G.R. (1966) The visual world of infants, in *The Nature and Nurture of Behaviour: Developmental Psychology. Readings from Scientific American* (ed. T. Greenough), Freeman & Co, San Francisco.

Bowlby, J. (1951) *Maternal Care and Mental health*, World Health Organization, Geneva.

Carpenter, G. (1974) Mothers' face and the newborn. *New Scientist*, **61** (890), 742–4.

Clarke, A.M. and Clarke, A.D.B. (1976) *Early Experience: Myth and Evidence*, Open Books, London.

Consumers' Association (1980) *Children in Hospital*, Consumers' Association, London.

Consumers' Association (1985) *Children in Hospital*, Consumers' Association, London.

Court, S.D.M. (1976) *Fit for the Future: Report of the Committee on Child Health Services, Volumes I and II*, HMSO, London.

Deater-Deckard, K., Pinkerton, R. and Scarr, S. (1996) Child Care Quality and Children's Behavioral Adjustment: a Four-Year Longitudinal Study. *Journal of Child Psychology and Psychiatry*, 37(8), 937–48.

Department of Health (1989) *The Children Act*, HMSO, London.

Department of Health (1991) *Welfare of Children and Young People in Hospital*, HMSO, London.

Department of Health (1996) *Child Health in the Community: a Guide to Good Practice*, Department of Health, London.

Douglas, J.W.B. (1975) Early hospital admissions and later disturbances of behaviour and learning. *Developmental Medicine and Child Neurology*, **17**, 456–80.

House of Commons (1997a) *Health Services for Children and Young People: Home and School. House of Commons Health Committee Third Report*, HMSO, London.

House of Commons (1997b) *The Specific Health Needs of Children and Young People. House of Commons Health Select Committee Second Report* HMSO, London.

Kagan, J., Kearsley, R.B. and Zelazo, P.R. (1978) *Infancy: Its Place in Human Development*, Harvard University Press, Cambridge, Massachusetts.

Lamb, M.E. (1981) *The Role of the Father in Child Development, 2nd edn*. John Wiley, New York.

Leidloff, J. (1978) *The Continuum Concept*, Futura, London.

Levy-Shiff, R. (1983) Adaptation and competence in early childhood: communally raised kibbutz children versus family raised children in the city. *Child Development*, **54**, 1606–14.

Platt, H. (1959) *The Welfare of Children in Hospital: Report of the Committee on Child Health Services*, HMSO, London.

Robertson, J. and Robertson, J. (1989) *Separation and the Very Young*, Free Association Books, London.

Rutter, M. (1975) Parent-child separation: psychological effects on children, in *Early Experience: Myth and Evidence* (eds A.M. Clarke and A.D.B. Clarke, 1976), Open Books, London.

Schaffer, H.R. (1977) *Mothering*, Fontana/Open Books, London.

Schaffer, H.R. (1990) *Making Decisions about Children*, Basil Blackwell, Oxford.

Sunley, R. (1955) Early nineteenth-century American literature on childrearing, in *Childhood in Contemporary Cultures* (eds M. Mead and M. Wolfenstein), University of Chicago Press, Chicago.

Thomas, S. (1994) Child's Play. *Nursing Times*, **90**(3), 43.

Wattley, L.A. and Müller, D.J. (1984) *Investigating Psychology: A Practical Approach for Nursing*, Harper & Row, London.

Wolkind, S. and Rutter, M. (1985) Separation, loss and family relationships, in *Child and Adolescent Psychiatry* (eds M. Rutter and L. Hersov), Blackwell Scientific Publications, Oxford.

Woodman, A. *1950s Sunday Express Baby Book*, Sunday Express, London.

World Health Organization (1951) *Expert Committee on Mental Health, Report on the Second Session 1951*, Technical Report Series No 31, WHO, Geneva.

FURTHER READING

Dimond, B. (1996) *The Legal Aspects of Child Health Care*, Mosby, London.
This excellent book provides information on current law, codes and charters and provides practical application through the examination of examples.

Hill Beuf, A. (1989) *Biting Off the Bracelet*, 2nd edn, University of Pennsylvania Press, Philadelphia.
This American text offers insight into the social care of children in hospital.

Maccoby, E.E. (1980) *Social Development. Psychological Growth and the Parent–Child Relationship*, Harcourt Brace, New York.

The early chapters trace the history of views on children and their rearing in more detail than is possible in our book, and then develop the theme of social development in relation to current knowledge and implications. Sample chapter titles are 'The sense of self'; 'Children's aggression and parental response'; 'Impulse control'.

Taylor, J. and Woods, M. (eds) *Early Childhood Studies: an Holistic Introduction*, Arnold, London.

This book, which takes a fresh approach to the study of children, explores the care of children from a number of perspectives including health, education and social care.

2 PSYCHOLOGY AND EARLY DEVELOPMENT

In our society childbirth takes place almost exclusively in a hospital setting with a major trend, over the last 20 years, away from home births (Kelnar, Harvey and Simpson, 1995). Some infants are treated further in special care nurseries or intensive care units, a number of which may employ few trained children's nurses or midwifery staff. Before reaching the age of 1 year, almost all babies will have spent some time in hospital, either healthy or sick, as in- or outpatients. Additionally, for various reasons, some will be re-admitted subsequently to paediatric units. This means that many health care professionals such as midwives, nursery nurses, student nurses, qualified nurses and health visitors will be concerned with the principles which underlie the psychological care of infants in hospital. Because of their contact with parents and others, these staff are in an ideal position to influence the care of infants after discharge. However, if infants are unable to tell us about their early experiences, how can we decide what principles are important in their care? To begin to try and answer this question, we need to investigate the implications of infancy.

INFANCY

Infancy is a period of time which can be thought of as the basis for later development, rather like the foundations that determine the ultimate shape and soundness of a building which are buried and are out of sight by the time the building is complete. Some would argue that this view fails to give sufficient prominence to demonstrate the psychological significance of infancy itself (e.g. Stratton, 1982) and may, in any case, be inaccurate (Karmiloff-Smith, 1995). In other words, although it is popular to think of evaluating early experience in terms of later outcomes (Chapter 1), it is equally important to appreciate the sophistication of infants in their own right. Stratton (1982) suggests that 'the perspective which sees babies as merely potential adults is misleading and fails to recognize the intrinsic value of the newborn' (p. 5). He gives examples of infant behaviours which are typically interpreted as preparation for maturity. For example, the early stepping and walking reflexes seen only in the first few days after birth which are often thought of as precursors to real walking (Figure 2.1). However this does not adequately explain why such reflexes fade long before real walking starts. An alternative explanation is that these reflexes merely facilitate the adoption of the vertex position before birth. Stratton proposes that infants can have experiences which can be 'valued in their own terms and without reference to any future consequences'.

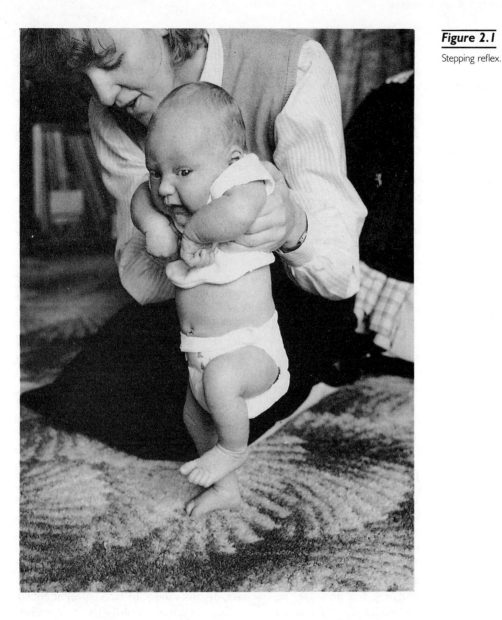

Figure 2.1

Stepping reflex.

If we take this view seriously when considering our approach to the care of infants in hospital, it is clear that the quality of an infant's experience matters just as much as the potential quality of his or her future life, especially as this is a time when it is difficult to assess the effect an experience has on the infant's physiological and psychological make-up. For example, infants feel pain, at least many of them scream and try to withdraw from a painful event such as having a blood sample taken. However, circumcision is performed on infant boys quite often without anaesthetic. Marshall (1989) reports that such experiences affect the infant at the time, both physiologically and psychologically (i.e. mother–infant interaction, crying and behaviour), but we do not know what, if any, are the long term effects of painful procedures (Carter, 1994). It would seem reasonable to establish that our habits in medical and nursing care minimize the risk of a painful introduction to early life, whether or not the effects can be shown to be long lasting.

In this chapter we are going to look at what is known about the development of infants during the first year of life. But when exactly does the first year of life begin? This is an important consideration because if we think of the birth as a beginning, we may be disregarding earlier factors which exert effects on the infant and the mother. Studies of antenatal psychology have, however, been limited not least because of the methodological difficulties involved. The mother and fetus have been viewed more as a biological than a psychological relationship, hence much of the research relates more to physical aspects of the relationship. For example, health education has tried to make mothers aware of the dangers of smoking, poor diet and drugs on the fetus, but less well known are those studies that have shown links between fears and worries on the part of the mother during pregnancy, and length of labour, analgesia requirements, and subsequent infant behaviour. Yang (1981) gives a detailed and very interesting consideration of this topic.

Our discussion starts with the development in the prenatal period and the reader might like to speculate on the question of when an embryo or fetus becomes a psychological being as the way this is viewed will presumably affect, in some way, the approach to the care of the mother during the antenatal period. This is also a well known ethical issue for nurses and midwives concerned with abortion and *in vitro* fertilization.

BEFORE BIRTH

Various behaviours occur in the antenatal period which resemble those needed to assist survival in the outside world. For example, from as early as 12 weeks after conception when fetuses are recognizably human, they can withdraw from irritants stimulating areas of the skin surface. They can also make sucking movements, if the mouth is touched, which mirror the spontaneous sucking of newborns in response to a nipple touching the lips. The significance of this ability to suck spontaneously can easily be overlooked. How many infants would survive if nurses actually had to teach all of them to suck as soon as they were born? As they grow a little older, fetuses will suck their thumbs and grasp the umbilical cord, which is just the right sort of size for them to do this. Nilsson (1980) describes the skills most needed by the newborn as 'suck, grasp and cling' and has demonstrated with photography the presence of these abilities *in utero*. Figure 2.2 shows a fetus at $4\frac{1}{2}$ months sucking its thumb, and Figure 2.3 shows a $5\frac{1}{2}$ month fetus grasping the umbilical cord.

In the uterus the fetus makes many types of movements from toe-curling and fanning, to kicking and making fists. By the end of the fourth month most mothers can begin to feel some movements. Before birth,

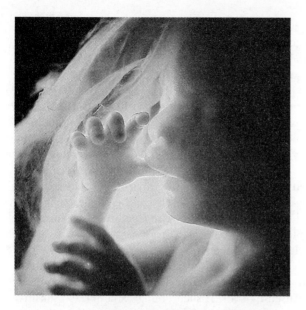

Figure 2.2

Fetus (4½ months old) sucking thumb. Reproduced with kind permission of the publishers from Nilsson (1980) *A Child is Born*, Faber and Faber, London.

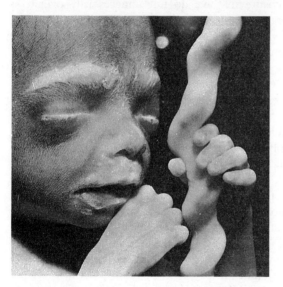

Figure 2.3

Fetus (5½ months old) grasping the umbilical cord. Reproduced by kind permission of the publishers from Nilsson (1980) *A Child is Born*, Faber and Faber, London.

fetuses have a startle reflex and they will sometimes demonstrate this in response to sudden loud sounds such as a door slamming. This suggests that the sense of hearing is present. Early experiments showed that the fetuses were not just responding to the mother's own reaction to sound, since they responded even if the mother was prevented from hearing an experimental sound by wearing headphones (MacFarlane, 1977). More recent experiments have demonstrated that the fetus can differentiate between sounds such as music and language. The fetus is also able to hear the mother's voice *in utero* and learn its sound to the extent that after birth the newborn infant can recognize and differentiate between the mother's voice and other female voices (Karmiloff-Smith, 1995). This is quite extraordinary given that sounds such as voices heard *in utero* are filtered through amniotic fluid which produces a 'muffling' effect.

We can also witness the presence of hearing in babies born prematurely by watching their reactions to sudden sounds. However, in these immature infants, sensitivity to sound appears to be manifested in more ways than just through the startle reflex. Morris (1994) reports research studies showing that preterm infants who have a planned programme of play which includes being talked to while in hospital will grow faster, have fewer respiratory problems, feed better and seem to develop better than babies not given this extra auditory stimulation. Researchers have for some time turned their attention to the environment surrounding babies in special care units, where noise levels can be dangerously high. Kelnar *et al.* (1995) discuss that the mean noise level inside an incubator should not exceed 60 decibels, but many routine noises such as the incubator alarm or closing the incubator door can exceed this. Wolke (1987), in his paper about neonatal special care units, also discusses sources of noise and recommended safety levels. He notes that 'noise pollution' is mainly caused by staff. If such young babies are so sensitive to sound, we need to ensure that we do not unnecessarily overstress their developing sense organs.

The development of vision takes place mainly after delivery. For the middle third of the pregnancy, the fetus's eyes are fused shut (Fig. 2.3). There is some sensitivity to light in the last three months before birth, when the eyelids open. Before birth the sensitivity is mainly unstimulated because light can only really penetrate if the mother's abdomen is taut due to the increasing size of the infant and if, for example, she sunbathes. However, babies born prematurely do demonstrate sensitivity to light, and this has implications for their care in neonatal units where it was habitual to have bright lights left on day and night to enable observation to be maintained, or where eye patches are used to protect the eyes for phototherapy in the treatment of jaundice, thus preventing visual input. There is now a greater awareness of the need to reduce noise and light stimulus at night (Kelnar *et al.*, 1995), although a longitudinal study by Wolke *et al.* (1995) found that the long term effects of being in a neonatal unit in relation to, for example, the incidence of later sleep disorders were not significant.

At birth, full-term infants have normally developed a range of sensory capacities which will help improve their chances of survival. In addition, these infants demonstrate a large number of reflexes in response to different stimuli including for example, grasping with both hands and the feet; stepping out as though walking if held upright above the surface, although just in contact with it; rooting towards the breast when touched on the cheek; sucking; eyeblinking; and reacting to sudden noise or changes in position by throwing back the arms and fanning the fingers (the Moro reflex, see Figure 2.4) as if to clutch at something for security. These reflexes and abilities are clearly illustrated and described in Illingworth (1987), who also discusses the differences between preterm and full-term babies.

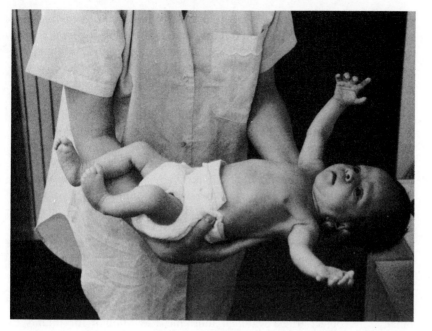

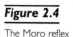

Figure 2.4

The Moro reflex

There is also a very brief summary of newborn capacities in Sheridan *et al.* (1997) followed by a valuable and detailed description of developmental progress over the first five years. Sheridan has used simple line drawings to illustrate various abilities and reflexes which are very effective for enabling the reader to recognize the developmental progress of babies.

We will now look at the psychological development of infants in more detail.

COMPETENT NEWBORNS

Vision

At birth, or shortly afterwards, it is possible to see evidence of the senses mentioned in the previous section. The most fascinating is sight. Fetuses before birth have probably never 'seen' anything with the exception of light and darkness (Karmiloff-Smith, 1995), yet once born and even before the cord has been cut, if held in an appropriate position infants can engage in mutual eye contact with another person. The position is called *en face* which means that an adult and infant are aligned with their faces in the same plane. The infant has a more or less fixed ideal focal length at this period which is about 20 centimetres and this corresponds well to the distance between the infant and a breastfeeding mother's face. It can also be achieved by people who bottlefeed, including nurses. In this sort of position infants can hold their gaze on the adult's eyes. Interestingly the infant's eyes can be particularly evocative for the parents. In early studies by MacFarlane (1977) it was noted that the baby's eyes seemed particularly important to the mothers because if they weren't open the mothers would often ask the infants to open them. For one mother the baby opening its eyes was the signal for her to greet it with 'Hello'. There are many anecdotal references to this sort of behaviour, which suggest that parents perceive the person as being in some way revealed through the eyes. Klaus and Kennell (1983) noted that the parents' affection and enthusiasm are stimulated and sustained by seeing the baby's open eyes. This is something the nurse can observe and discuss with parents.

It is not at all uncommon to find parents (and nurses) who still believe that infants are born blind like baby rats or kittens. What is needed is for them to observe a newborn baby under the right conditions. For about an hour after birth many babies are quietly alert, but after this time they sleep a lot and may only manage quiet alertness occasionally in the next few days. However, they need to be in this quiet alert state to demonstrate their visual capacities. Secondly, unless they are supported appropriately, they cannot coordinate their responses to stimuli. New babies lying flat on their backs can only balance by using their heads and limbs so it is difficult for them to watch a moving object. Finally, the object to be watched must be slow enough for infants to coordinate their muscles. Under these conditions, which amount to holding the alert infant well supported and slowly moving an object across the field of vision which is about eight inches from the eyes, it should be obvious that the infant can see.

Infants seem particularly attracted to high contrast moving objects, so a child's bright red brick would be an ideal object, but of course human eyes are high contrast moving objects within the face, with sharply defined white and dark areas which catch the light. The infant therefore can find quite accidentally and unintentionally a rewarding object in the environment which also rewards the parents for whom eye contact seems to be especially important. It may help develop the strong emotional commitment or bond which will enable them to care for the infant under circumstances which are often going to be stressful, prolonged and exhausting.

Hearing

Babies can hear when they are born, although, after birth, sounds are muted for a few days until fluid is absorbed from within the ear. Rhythmic sounds will have surrounded the baby in the uterus for many months, the mother's heartbeat and bowel sounds being the most common. It is hardly surprising, then, that a metronome or other rhythmic sound paced like a heartbeat is meaningful to an infant. Singing, the radio and even the vacuum cleaner have been discovered by mothers to soothe or excite babies. Haith (1986) reports experiments which have investigated hearing in newborns and show that they can localize sound sources by turning or looking towards the source. Other studies discussed by Haith noted changes in heart rate, respiration and muscle tension in response to sound. Some researchers found that infants are more attentive to sounds with a large frequency variation. It is interesting to note that observations of human verbal interactions with babies show that, typically, they use a wide variety of frequency.

Touch and proprioception

We have already mentioned that babies react to pain. They also have more subtle tactile sensitivities. They often cry if clothing is removed, and will swipe at irritants such as cotton wool tickling a part of their body. Even preterm babies are susceptible to tactile stimulation. Klaus and Kennell (1983) reviewed several research studies of preterm infants which showed that premature infants who are touched, rocked, fondled or cuddled daily showed faster development and gained more weight than babies not receiving extra stimulation. Whitelaw *et al.* (1988) also showed that, when mothers were encouraged to have skin to skin contact with their very low birthweight infants, they lactated for longer and babies cried for significantly shorter periods. The ability to swipe fairly accurately at irritants suggests the presence of another sensory capacity called proprioception. This is the sense which tells us where our limbs are even if we cannot see them. It is achieved by registering the angles of bones within joints though we are not conscious of our skill except perhaps when injury causes it to fail, as in patients who suffer paralysis after a cerebrovascular accident. They may have to be taught to look at their limbs in order to see if they are positioned appropriately.

Taste and smell

It is also possible to demonstrate that babies have sense of smell and of taste. For example, if presented with a breast pad from their own mother and a clean one they will spend more time facing towards their mother's: similarly they will turn towards their own mother's pad in preference to an unfamiliar mother's (MacFarlane, 1977). Other studies have shown that they will turn away from a noxious smell (Haith, 1986). Weiffenbach (in Mussen *et al.*, 1990) in a study of 175 babies, photographed their responses when given lemon juice and sugar solutions to taste. Results showed that babies preferred the sugar solution and responded in a similar way to adults when given lemon juice.

All these sensory capacities are impressive as examples of infant competence, but they are not simply manifestations of infants' passive reactions to their world. They contribute to enable the infant to mobilize the means for survival. Infants need to be able to attract attention for caregiving activities such as feeding, cuddling and changing in order to survive, and to establish a bond with a caregiver which will ensure that care is forthcoming in the future. If they can achieve this, they also have the opportunity to develop physically and psychologically and this requires appropriate experiences and levels of stimulation.

In the next section we will explore the relationship between infants and the external environment. One of the fascinating aspects of this relationship which will be evident is the active role played by the infant in obtaining opportunities for learning and development.

UNDERSTANDING THE ENVIRONMENT

Even at birth it is possible to demonstrate that infants possess the sophisticated raw materials in sensory terms which will enable them to begin to exert some control over the environment. At first this may only be in a very minimal way, for example by shutting their eyes to reduce visual stimulation when light is too bright, turning away from sounds or smells, or swiping at irritants on the body. Even these sensory capacities are going to change because infants keep on growing. The significance of this is that infants presumably have to continue modifying their relationship to the world. As the body increases in size, so the sense organs must accommodate changes in the way the world is perceived. The ears and the eyes grow further apart as the head grows, the skin surface increases in area, and the limbs grow longer so that tactile capacities must accommodate altered messages. Since babies grow very rapidly one might assume that they would be continuously confused by the constant need to adapt to their sensory world. It is interesting that this is far from the case. For example, if babies see an object and want to reach out and grasp it, they need accurate hand–eye coordination. If they do not have this or maintain it as they grow they will have great difficulty in reaching objects accurately until they stop growing. However, it is clear from observing infants that they are in fact quite accurate on most occasions, whilst toddlers rarely misjudge the location of an object, although they too are still growing.

Bower (1977) explains this behaviour by referring to infants as young as 2 weeks old, when they can be seen catching sight of their own hands as they are waved into their visual field. Infants may repeatedly interrupt a reaching movement for an object to gaze intently at their hands. After a number of these interruptions, called 'hand-regard', the infants appear to become used to their own hands and Bower (1977) proposes that they then use them by comparing the hands which they can see approaching the object with the object itself. Thus, they can make fine adjustments by relating the hand, the object and the distance between them and reach to grasp the object with accuracy.

In learning to make accurate grasping movements for objects, infants are making complicated adjustments of hand and eye, and learning to organize sensory capacities to make sense of the world. However, these capacities do not function in isolation, and it is doubtful whether infants really distinguish between them, since in the early months they will look towards a sound (as if expecting to see something) and reach towards a visible object (as if expecting to touch it), rather than applying one sense to one particular stimulus. The ability to locate a sound source is also interesting because infants seem to show distress if they are unable to make sense of a particular auditory experience. Bower (1982) describes an experimental situation in which infants were positioned opposite a glass soundproof screen through which they could see their mother. The mother's voice was relayed to the infant through speakers, which could manipulate the voice to make it sound as though the sound source was not from the mother at all, but somewhere to the left or right. Infants as young as 3 weeks old were disturbed by this, and appeared to have learned already that a voice should come from a mouth.

Results like these are of great interest and are obviously exciting, but it is always wise to be cautious with this kind of material, and to remain open-minded to alternative explanations. For example, Bower mentions criticisms about the conclusion that infants were distressed by the disassociation of mother and voice. An alternative explanation is that they were distressed by trying to orientate to two sources of stimuli, a visual one (the mother) and an auditory one (the speakers), positioned in different places. However, the point remains that infant behaviour can be seen to be organized, and not be a random confusion of experiences.

These examples illustrate a degree of organization in very young infants' responses to the stimuli around them. Although the organization may be something of which infants themselves are unconscious, it is apparent that they are rather less confused by their experiences than we might imagine. There is a degree of selectivity in the organization of infant behaviour. For example, newborns are particularly responsive to higher pitched (usually female) voices (Mussen *et al.*, 1990), and to certain visual features in the environment particularly those features with patterns and contours (Haith, 1986; Karmiloff-Smith, 1995). The ability of babies to, for instance, attend to visual objects will affect their ability to react and in the first few weeks, the infant seems only able to pay attention to parts of objects. It is well known that by 6 weeks the infant will smile at human faces. However, initially, the complete face is not necessary to elicit the smiling reaction and all that is required are marks like eyes or lines like lips. However, it appears to be important to the newborn infant that these marks are arranged in a face-like configuration. Johnson and Morton (1991) did some detailed experiments showing that, even within the first hour of life, newborn babies show preference to a configuration which mimics the human face (i.e. two dark squares in the place of eyes, above one dark square in the place of the mouth), rather than a configuration with scrambled features or one with one dark square above two dark squares. Johnson and Morton do warn about drawing conclusions from these data. 'That is not to say, however, that neonates have any conception of the meaning of a face. All that can be said is that they prefer to track a pattern that has face-like properties' (p. 106).

In addition to studying the particular aspects of the environment to which babies attend, it is possible to investigate whether babies can exercise choices over the things to which they attend. Karmiloff-Smith (1995) discusses studies that have looked at visual discrimination. She cites one study which found that some babies of only 4 days old can discriminate between their mother's face and the faces of strangers. It appears that the infant differentiates by focusing on the face/hairline and the outer contour of the mother's head. According to Karmiloff-Smith infants can become quite distressed if a mother drastically changes her hairstyle! By 2 months the infant will start to focus on the actual face and Wolkind and Rutter (1985) suggest that infants discriminate consistently by 3 months. Kaye (1982) warns, however, that studies have not always accounted for differences in behaviour between mothers and strangers.

Another example of the sophisticated nature of babies' powers of organization is the ability of babies of only a few weeks old, who have never seen their own face, to imitate the gesture of poking out the tongue. This means the infant has to pick out the right section of the experimenter's face, recognize the existence of the tongue, recognize their own tongues (which they cannot compare with the experimenter's because they can only feel, not see it) and coordinate the muscles needed to poke their own out of their mouths (Vinter, 1986). An interesting study by Meltzoff and Moore (1994) elaborated on this theme by presenting a group of 6 week old babies with an adult who repeatedly stuck his tongue out. The next day the babies were again presented with the same adult who kept his mouth closed. After observing the adult's face the babies proceeded to stick out their tongues. They did not elicit this response when presented with a different adult.

Research suggests then that an infant's senses are all functional to varying degrees. Haith (1986, p. 68) concludes:

Even at birth, babies are much more than recipients of environmental stimuli. They possess action systems for deploying their sensory and perceptual apparatus for discovering, selecting and analysing aspects of the world around them.

It appears then that most babies follow a fairly predictable pattern of motor and perceptual development during the first year of life. This is the stage that Piaget referred to as 'sensori-motor' (Chapter 4) and is characterized by the need for infants to learn by doing. If they cannot experience the environment through touching, sucking and so on, it is thought that they cannot develop properly. The point is that the brain has to function in order to develop appropriately. Thus, some babies who, for whatever reason, are not afforded opportunities and experiences, such as those identified by Super (1987) in cross-cultural studies into infant development, may show relative developmental delay. Meerum Terwogt *et al.* (1990) found that developmental delay persists even among children of school age.

THE ROLE OF CARERS

Research relating to the principles of early experience and their effects on intellectual and social development has been reviewed by Schaffer (1990) and Mussen *et al.* (1990). The single most important factor for the infant's optimum development seems to be the caregiver's responsiveness to the infant. It is thought that this helps infants to learn that they can have an effect on their environment, which in turn can help later on in the development of reasoning powers. The nature of the caregiver's responsiveness is important in that variety, intensity and frequency of stimulation all seem to be closely related to the child's development, and different children require different degrees of stimulation. Another very important factor is the appropriateness of the stimulation provided for the particular child. Too much, or too complex stimulation can cause problems. The importance of quality of stimulation and responsiveness of the caregiver to an individual child seems to suggest that the optimum role of the caregiver is not purely directive, but based on sensitivity to the infant's needs.

Most of the research studies in this field are concerned with mothers, and therefore it can appear that only mothers can fulfil the role of caregiving, though this may be a problem arising from the nature of the research. Other people (e.g. father, friend, grandparent) can develop responsiveness and sensitivity to individual children, and nurses too can aim to achieve this by organizing their caregiving around a few individual children rather than all sharing all the tasks to be done in one ward. Brown (1989), in her study of individualized care compared with task allocation on two children's wards, demonstrated the benefits to children and their families when individualized care was practised. Nurses are more likely to recognize and respond to needs, other than obvious physical needs, if they are able to build up a relationship with the child and family.

It has been said that nursing aims to maintain optimum physiological and psychological functioning in patients. If this is a real aim, dare we ignore the research describing the importance of responsiveness to the individual infant for optimum psychological development? In the first year of life, the type of stimulation which seems to be most associated with mental development is physical, including cuddling, carrying, playing and providing opportunities to move about and test out the environment. Towards the end of the first year this is superseded by verbal stimulation, corresponding with the beginning of language development.

So far we have talked almost exclusively about the capacities of infants, but have mentioned only briefly the potential significance of sensitive and responsive caregivers. If the infant's development is really so dependent on the relationship established with the caregiver, then the infant's social contexts should also be observed. Babies cannot survive in isolation from a caregiver. Infants' development then is closely linked with other people.

BECOMING SOCIAL

Some people believe that infants are born social, while others feel that the potential is there and develops gradually along with other characteristics. Socialization is the name given to the process by which a child becomes integrated into society 'by adopting its norms and values, acquiring the necessary skills of social interaction, and learning to adopt an acceptable role' (Stratton and Hayes, 1993, p. 188). If we look at infant behaviour only in terms of the 'process' described here, we may fail to appreciate an infant's behaviour in the 'here and now', whereas infants engage in behaviours that provoke social interaction from the first day of life, even though they may have no conscious intention of being sociable.

As mentioned above, a neonate can make eye contact with another person within seconds of delivery. If a mother has time with her infant, then she may respond in a fairly predictable way (MacFarlane, 1977; Klaus and Kennell, 1982). For example, initially the mother will probably use her fingertips to explore the infant's own tiny fingers and nails; she may tentatively find and touch its feet and gradually begin to caress its body. MacFarlane (1997) was struck in his early studies by the richness, complexity and passion of the first encounters, but also by how disruptive obstetric procedures such as suturing, delivery of the placenta and wrapping the baby up were. Sleep (1995) suggests that the midwife should safeguard the first precious moments after birth which are moments 'to be savoured and treasured' (p. 132) even if only for a few precious moments. This is of great importance to the development of the mother–child relationship. A study by Ball (1994) found, for example, that maternal satisfaction with 'motherhood' at 6 weeks was closely linked to feelings immediately after birth and to being able to feed the baby within the first hour.

In contrast, where a baby was sick and in an incubator, Klaus and Kennell (1982) noted a difficulty for mothers in getting past the fingertip-touching stage. Their research into the nature of bonding arose from this observation, and has led to the realization by hospitals that parents need help to overcome their awe of the institution and form a relationship with their own baby. Kelnar et al. (1995) suggest that all parents should at least see, and ideally cuddle their baby before transfer to a neonatal unit. Instant photographs should be taken and given to the parents and if the baby has to be transferred to a distant unit ideally the mother should go too. 'Bonding' is the term given to a one-way process from parent to child, which is recognized to be occurring by certain types of behaviour such as fondling, kissing, cuddling, talking and prolonged gazing. The behaviours usually seem to happen, despite the absence of any sign of affection from the infant at this stage.

When the theories of bonding first began to affect hospital attitudes about the early hours after delivery, there was sometimes an unfortunate effect from overstating the significance of early interaction, which consequently led to parents feeling guilty, or failures, if something prevented them from making the appropriate overtures to their infant. Previous experience, home backgrounds as well as beliefs and attitudes all contribute to the complexity of factors which can exert effects on early parent–infant interaction and we are now able to view the process of bonding with greater flexibility. Increasingly, hospitals are relaxing their attitudes and trying to respond on an individual basis to the needs of families in this respect. Bonding is not something which can be prescribed. In many ways it resembles the private development of a courtship between two adults, and will need to form in its own way for each family.

One of the noticeable things about many early encounters is the way the parents ascribe to the baby individual characteristics (father's nose, mother's temper, etc.). People seem to expect the infant to have certain personality characteristics and all of us will have heard comments such as 'Why are you looking so cross?' or 'What's worrying you?' or 'You look as though you've been here before', implying a degree of knowledge of the world. Adults seem to be looking for (or is it responding to?) aspects of infants as if they are unique, with their own personality and individuality.

Babies seem to be very good at attracting adults. Their 'babyness' has been copied by Walt Disney to make particular characters attractive, such as 'Bambi', whose big head, jerky movements and domed forehead are not unlike the features of many newborns. These and other characteristics seem to stimulate a response in the parents to want to care for the infant. Although some early features of babies' behaviour and appearance may promote caring attitudes in the parents, it is still possible for parents to forget sometimes that they have a baby at all, and from time to time babies get left accidentally on buses or in shops. This may be because in the West we tend to parcel up babies separately from the parents, in carrycots and prams. In some other societies the baby rarely leaves the mother's body as they are tied on with slings, and it is reported that in these societies the infants do not necessarily signal their needs by crying, except in emergencies. Instead the mothers seem to respond to particular movements made by the baby (Greenfield, cited by Bee, 1997). In our society it is fortunate that babies can cry to signal their needs if they are going to be kept separate from parents who will therefore be unable to see or feel their condition. The newborn's cry is particularly irritating to adults, which seems to be a good way of ensuring that they react quickly to it. It is interesting that a study by Whitelaw *et al.* (1988) in London, which encouraged mothers to carry their low birthweight infants next to their skin, head up between their breasts (in what is described as 'Kangaroo' baby care), resulted in the mothers lactating for longer and the babies crying less (see also Sleath, 1994).

Crying

Babies cry for a number of reasons. Initially crying is a response to sensations within or around the baby such as cold, hunger, or other forms of discomfort. We have already seen how babies learn rapidly to associate particular sensory experiences and to control them (e.g. ignoring a stranger but looking at their mother). Infants' capacity for learning is impressive, and it gradually affects their crying patterns. When babies cry they tend to receive a cuddle, food, or a change of clothes, and so they learn that cries bring certain responses. Armed with this knowledge, infants are now able to employ crying as a conscious signal to achieve desired goals. One early experiment described by Bower (1977) ingeniously revealed the learning capacities of the newborn. The experimenter used apparatus which, if the newborn turned its head to the right at the sound of a tone, delivered a sweet-tasting solution to the infant's mouth. If a buzzer sounded and the infant turned its head to the left, it could also receive the solution. After only a few trials the newborns turned correctly to the right when the tone sounded and to the left for the buzzer. If newborns can demonstrate this ability to learn so fast then it is hardly surprising if learning occurs in relation to crying over the next few weeks.

In the experiment by Bower (1977), the learning was reinforced by the sweet-tasting solution. This pleasant taste is similar to the reward of a cuddle or food and thus babies are reinforced in their learning about the consequences of crying.

Crying and distress in infants can cause parents (and nurses) great problems, especially when they cannot find the cause or stop the noise. There are great individual differences between babies and the amount they grizzle, cry and fret. Some babies are more cuddly than others, and in one interesting research finding described by Dunn (1977) it was found that if a mother had an anaesthetic during labour, the infant was more likely to be irritable. Dunn also found that babies born after long deliveries cried more and slept less, but the causal relationship is difficult to establish. Maternal anxiety is linked with longer labour and more drugs, but it could also be said that the antenatal anxiety had affected the child in the uterus, rather than the specific effects of the labour or the drugs. Such questions are very difficult to resolve, but it may be consoling for some mothers who have had difficult labours to understand that many babies are difficult to settle after this sort of experience.

Over the course of the first year the causes of crying modify from reactions to hunger, pain, cold exposure and sudden changes in stimulation, to include responses to teasing, frustration, strangers, and fear or anxiety. Part of the reason for these changes relates to the infant's ability to identify and miss the primary caregiver. Many infants develop a special attachment to a 'comforter' such as a piece of soft cloth, and this substitute seems to induce calmness during the second half of the first year until much later into childhood (Rutter and Cox, 1985). Sparshott (1994) gives an excellent account of the causes of distress in infants and the means of comfort, which could be particularly helpful to nurses. Fortunately for adults, crying is not an infant's only means of communication.

Smiling

One of the most exciting and rewarding behaviours that parents enjoy with their baby in the first few weeks is the smile. As already described, as infants' capacity for attention increases, they smile at more complete images of human faces. Though in the first few weeks of life, there are fleeting smiles (often associated with wind), the smile is thought not to occur until 3–6 weeks after delivery. This true smile involves the whole face, lighting up the eyes in a very attractive way, and is seen in relation to particular sights and sounds. Human faces and voices in particular seem to cause smiling to occur. By 3 months of age the infant will have learnt, as with crying, to produce a smile in order to get a response from, say, the mother.

Psychologists have speculated on the meaning of the smile and why, if it is so rewarding a behaviour, it does not occur fully until some weeks after delivery. One view is that this is a survival mechanism evolved from the days when maternal and perinatal mortality rates were very high. One early theory is that if the natural mothers should die, then substitutes can still experience great reinforcement from the infants to care for them, and infants can therefore develop an interaction with someone other than the mother (MacFarlane, 1974). This is a theory which would be very difficult to test, but ideas like this can be useful in helping us to consider why such behaviours have developed in human babies.

EARLY INTERACTION

There is another less obvious way in which infants contribute to their social development, which has been described in detail by Kaye (1982). By observing mothers feeding their infants, it is usually possible to note a pattern that looks rather like turn-taking. While the infant is sucking, mothers usually sit quietly looking at their infant, or perhaps reading, watching television, chatting or dozing. Infants tend to suck in bursts, interspersed with pauses. Mothers quite often unconsciously use the pauses as a signal to start jiggling the babies, talking to them, tickling their feet, pulling faces and engaging in mutual gaze. Some of the time this may be to stimulate the infants to complete the feeds. As soon as they start to suck again the mothers stop and sit quietly. It appears that mothers slot their activity into the appropriate places in response to their infants' own pattern of behaviour.

Kaye (1982) has referred to this turn-taking pattern between the mothers and the infants as part of learning the rules that govern turn-taking in adulthood. Initially, babies may be unaware of their turns and therefore the interaction is rather one-sided in that the mother's sensitivity determines the synchrony. Still, the exposure to communication patterns, by constant repetition, is likely to instil in infants a sense of the rules of communication long before any speech or language develops, and it is possible for infants to communicate at least some messages before saying a single word (see also Goldbart, 1988 for accounts of turn-taking in early infant play). The verbal stimulation encountered by the infant becomes increasingly significant towards the end of the first year but, despite this, it is not possible to prepare an infant verbally for an experience such as hospitalization. Concepts of time are still relatively meaningless, and the infant continues to experience the world from and through the relative safety and guidance of the caregivers.

The infant's attachment to the caregiver is a topic of some controversy because, as shown in Chapter 1, most of the research has concerned mothers and infants and gives the impression that attachment is unique to this relationship. Similarly, attachment is a difficult behaviour to measure, especially in preverbal infants. Attachment has been thought to be a vital factor in child development, which is often disrupted by hospitalization, and below we will consider the meaning and measurement of it.

Attachment

While 'bonding' is the term used to describe a parent's caring relationship to an infant, attachment has been used to describe the infant's particular relationship to significant others. Chapter 1 shows that this relationship is not limited to one caregiver. Attachment is not apparent at birth, it seems to develop over a period of time. Limitations in the infant's ability to communicate mean that it is very difficult to be sure when it has happened. A crude measure is that after a certain age, infants can get excited, or fret, about a particular person to whom they may cling if they anticipate being separated. At around the age of 6 months, though it varies from infant to infant, babies seem to realize that people can disappear from view, and this may upset them. They have to learn that absence is usually temporary and that people still exist and can return, even if they cannot be seen at the time, and that when they return they are in fact the same person rather than a different one. An experiment described in Bower (1982) demonstrates how infants change in their understanding of these problems. Up to 5 months of age, infants shown multiple images of their mothers show no surprise and in fact may even seem rather pleased, interacting with all of them but, after 5 months, they become upset. If, however, the set of images consists of the mother and two strangers, the older infant interacts happily with the image of the mother and is not disturbed. Bower interprets this as showing that by now infants know they have only one mother, whereas when younger they thought they had several.

In the same experiment younger infants were also shown their mother and two strangers, and interacted with the mother just as the infants did in other studies. It is difficult to know whether these behaviours indicate attachment, though they do seem to indicate recognition. As babies become more mobile from about 7 months, they begin to search for objects that they have dropped and this searching can also be seen when infants can do something about keeping their caregivers nearby. They may make crude tugging or pushing movements which disrupt the caregiver's activity (e.g. snatching at a magazine or the telephone) and when they can crawl or walk they may follow the caregiver and stay within range. If passed to a stranger they may protest loudly and, if tired, hurt or ill, they will cling to the caregiver (usually the mother) in preference to others, which all seem to be examples of attachment behaviours.

The behaviour of children towards strangers changes at about the same time as their demonstration of attachment towards certain known individuals. Up to about 6 months of age, many infants do not protest at being close to strangers and will allow a degree of interaction. With the development of attachments they became more wary of strangers. In experiments described by Maccoby (1980), infants stayed closer to their mothers in the presence of strangers (even if the father was also present). However, if the mother remained nearby, the infants warmed to the strangers and began to play. If the mother left, the infants lost interest in the play and some cried. Some behaviour was described as 'suspended' as the children waited by the door for the mother's return, or sat immobile holding but not playing with a toy they had been involved with. These behaviours are especially marked in strange situations such as hospitals and clinics, but are much less obvious in the child's home.

Although we have said that attachment refers to the response of the child to particular important individuals, it is actually somewhat misleading to imply that it occurs irrespective of any factors in the object of the infant's attachment or indeed the child himself (Rutter, 1995). The development of secure attachment is related to features of the parents (and others) and their responsiveness as well as the child's own temperament. According to Dunn (1993) parents will, for example, have different relationships with different children. Several dimensions are important, among them being sensitivity – insensitivity, acceptance – rejection, cooperation – interference and accessibility – ignoring (Maccoby, 1980). Each of these dimensions represents a range along which people's behaviour may be positioned and, as a result, affect the attachment of the infant. Thus, there is a need to study infants in their social context if we are to build up a clear picture of their development.

As stated, from birth, infants must provoke someone to care for them. In so doing they mobilize the resources they need for physical and psychological development. They need not be confused and passive recipients of experience but, given sensitive caregivers, can explore the world in an ordered way and gradually begin to reciprocate and interact to form true relationships in a social context. They rapidly learn relationships between their own behaviours and specific consequences, and build on this knowledge to exert some control over their world and bring about desired goals. By the age of 1 year, infants are able to sit unsupported, crawl, stand and often walk. They can pick up tiny objects like string between finger and thumb, throw, find and retrieve toys, watch people and recognize familiar ones even at a distance. They respond immediately to their own name, babble in conversational tones and understand particular words and phrases, and carry out simple instructions, for example, to carry something or give an object to a particular person. They also demonstrate the use of particular items (Figure 2.5).

The complexity of infant development really demands further reading, especially for those who care specifically for this age group. Several themes emerge in the study of early development to serve as a useful guide to the subject matter.

Figure 2.5

Definition by use of everyday objects.

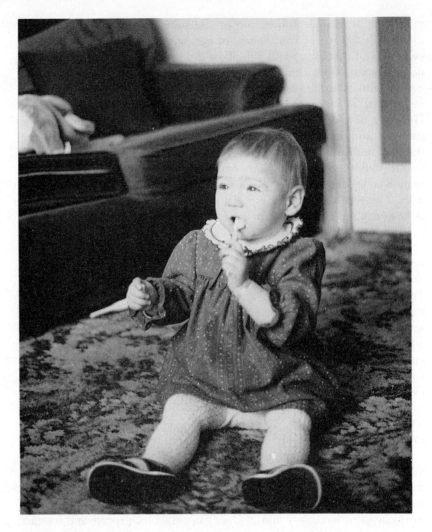

THEMES IN THE STUDY OF EARLY DEVELOPMENT

The first theme is the significance of infancy as a distinct period of time in its own right, rather than purely as a foundation period for later life. To take such an approach into account may mean that we have to ask ourselves about the values we place on the treatment and care of infants. It also demands that we acquire knowledge of the unique and specific behaviours of infancy.

A second important theme is the need to interpret infant behaviour in the context for which it was apparently designed. We can state with some certainty that it was not designed for hospitals. However, the infant clearly functions within a social context, and hospitals need not disrupt that. If given the chance, infants form attachments to a range of individuals. Most research concentrates on the mother–infant relationship because this is convenient, but this means that our picture of the infant's social world may actually be distorted.

A third theme concerns the difficulty of understanding the real needs of infants and of inferring their reactions to experiences from their behaviour. Since we cannot use words and language to warn infants about their world, we must rely on other means of optimizing their quality of life. One important principle is the significance of the primary caregiver, who is especially sensitive to the needs of the infant and can interpret the world appropriately for the infant by adjusting the variety, quantity and intensity of stimulation.

Finally an important development principle for infants in the first year is that in order to develop they need to be able actively to explore their world. This means that they need appropriate experiences to enable them to develop motor, coordination, perceptual and cognitive skills. Such skills are also vital in the development of social behaviour. Awareness of infants' active (as opposed to passive) roles in the development of understanding in their world, combined with knowledge of the parents' preparedness to sustain and develop an early and lasting relationship should help to make us sensitive to the environmental and social needs of the family unit and focus our attention on this rather than on the infant alone.

◄ *In practice*

- Infants need sensitive caregivers who respond appropriately to their individual needs for experience and stimulation. This suggests that one nurse or midwife should care for only a few infants and try to get to know them intimately.
- The presence of the normal caregiver helps the infant to explore new situations and cope with strangers. Parents and others should be made welcome and their importance to the infant acknowledged by the whole paediatric unit. It will help if staff clarify what parents can do and how they can be of practical assistance.
- Infants can only develop appropriately through physical experience of the environment and people around them. They need to hold, taste and suck things, to move about, experiment and learn. Ensuring that infants are able to obtain appropriate experience is a priority, not an optional luxury, and it is central to the nurse's role with infants.
- Infants form attachments to a variety of people, including parents. These relationships are important and must be taken into account so that the infant is not nursed in isolation from the family and any social network. Where infection risks might disrupt this, special planning may be needed.
- It is important that nursing personnel acknowledge the developing psychological relationship between mother and fetus, even before birth. Midwives should be encouraged to investigate the relationship between the mother's fears and worries in pregnancy and the subsequent experience of labour and mother–infant interaction.

REFERENCES

Ball, J. (1994) *Reactions to Motherhood: The role of post natal care*, 2nd edn, Books for Midwives Press, Cheshire.

Bee, H. (1997) *The Developing Child*, 8th edn, Longman, New York.

Bower, T.G.R. (1977) *A Primer of Infant Development*. W.H. Freeman, San Francisco.

Bower, T.G.R. (1982) *Development in Infancy*, 2nd edn, W.H. Freeman, San Francisco.

Brown, R. (1989) *Individualised Care*, Scutari Press, Middlesex.

Carter, B. (1994) *Child and Infant Pain: Principles of Nursing Care and Management*, Chapman and Hall, London.

Dunn, J. (1977) *Distress and Comfort*, Fontana: Open Books, London.

Dunn, J. (1993) *Young Children's Close Relationships: beyond attachment, Individual Differences and Development Series*, Vol. 4, Sage, Newbury Park.

Goldbart, J. (1988) Re-examining the Development of early Communication, in *Communication Before Speech*, (eds J. Coupe and J. Goldbart), Croom Helm, London.

Haith, M.M. (1986) Sensory and perceptual processes in early infancy. *Journal of Pediatrics*, **109**(19), 158–71.

Illingworth, R.S. (1987) *The Development of the Infant and Young Child*, 9th edn, Churchill Livingstone, Edinburgh.

Johnson, M.H. and Morton, J. (1991) *Biology and Cognitive Development: the case of face recognition*, Blackwell, Oxford.

Karmiloff-Smith, A. (1995) The extraordinary cognitive journey from foetus through infancy. *Journal of Child Psychology and Psychiatry*, **36**(8), 1293 – 1313.

Kaye, K. (1982) *The Mental and Social Life of Babies*, The University of Chicago Press, Chicago.

Kelnar, C.J.H., Harvey, D. and Simpson, C. (1995) *The Sick Newborn Baby*, 3rd edn, Baillière Tindall, London.

Klaus, M.H. and Kennell, J.H. (1982) *Parent–Infant Bonding*, Mosby, St Louis.

Klaus, M. and Kennell, J. (1983) An evaluation of interventions in the premature nursery, in *Parent–Baby Attachment in Premature Infants*, (eds J.A. Davis, M.P.M. Richards and N.R.C. Robertson), Croom Helm, London.

Maccoby, E.E. (1980) *Social Development: Psychological Growth and the Parent Child Relationship*, Harcourt Brace, New York.

MacFarlane, A. (1974) If a smile is so important. *New Scientist*, **62**(895), 164–6.

MacFarlane, A. (1977) *The Psychology of Childbirth*. Harvard University Press, Cambridge, Mass.

Marshall, R.E. (1989) Neonatal pain associated with caregiving procedures. *Pediatric Clinics of North America*, 36(4), 885–903.

Meerum Terwogt, M., Schene, J. and Koops, W. (1990) Concepts of emotion in institutionalized children. *Journal of Child Psychology and Psychiatry*, **31**(7), 1131–43.

Meltzoff, A.N. and Moore, M.K. (1994) Initiation, Memory and the Representation of Persons. *Infant Behaviour and Development*, 17, 83–99

Morris, M. (1994) Enhancing Development in the Neonatal Unit, in *Neonatal Nursing*, (eds D. Crawford and M. Morris), Chapman and Hall, London.

Mussen, P.H., Conger, J.J., Kagan, J. and Huston, A.C. (1990) *Child Development and Personality*, 7th edn, Addison Wesley, London.

Nilsson, L. (1980) *A Child is Born*, Faber & Faber, London.

Rutter, M. (1995) Clinical Implications of Attachment Concepts. *Journal of Child Psychology and Psychiatry*, **36**(4), 549–71.

Rutter, M. and Cox, A. (1985) Other family influences, in *Child and Adolescent Psychiatry*, (eds M. Rutter and L. Hersov), Blackwell Scientific Publications, Oxford.

Schaffer, H.R. (1990) *Making Decisions about Children*, Basil Blackwell, Oxford.

Sheridan, M.D., Frost, M. and Sharman, A. (1997) *From Birth to Five Years: Children's Developmental Progress*, 2nd edn, Routledge, London.

Sleath, K. (1994) Home Oxygenation, in *Neonatal Nursing*, (eds D. Crawford and M. Morris), Chapman and Hall, London.

Sleep, J. (1995) Postnatal Perineal Care Revisited, in *Aspects of Midwifery Practice: a research based approach*, (eds J. Alexander, V. Levy and S. Roch), Macmillan, Basingstoke.

Sparshott, M. (1994) Nursing Care of a Baby in Pain and Discomfort, in *Neonatal Nursing*, (eds D. Crawford and M. Morris), Chapman and Hall, London.

Stratton, P. (1982) *Psychobiology of the Human Newborn*, John Wiley, Chichester.

Stratton, P. and Hayes, N. (1993) *A Student's Dictionary of Psychology*, 2nd edn, Arnold, London.

Super, C.M. (1987) Cross-Cultural Research on Infancy, in *Cognitive Development in Infancy*, (eds J. Oates and S. Sheldon), Psychology Press, Hove.

Vinter, A. (1986) The role of movement in eliciting early imitations, *Child Development*, **57**, 66–71.

Whitelaw, A., Heisterkame, G., Sleath, K., Acolet, D. and Richards, M. (1988) Skin to skin contact for very low birth weight infants and their mothers. *Archives of Disease in Childhood*, **63**, 1377–81.

Wolke, D. (1987) Environmental neonatology. *Archives of Disease in Childhood*, **62**(10), 987–8.

Wolke, D., Meyer, R., Ohrt, B. and Riegel, K. (1995) The Incidence of Sleeping Problems in Pre-term and Full Term Infants Discharged from Neonatal Special Care Units: an epidemiological longitudinal study. *Journal of Child Psychology and Psychiatry*, **36**(2), 203–23.

Wolkind, S. and Rutter, M. (1985) Separation, loss and family relationships, *Child and Adolescent Psychiatry*, (eds M. Rutter and L. Hersov), Blackwell Scientific Publications, Oxford.

Yang, R.K. (1981) Maternal attitudes during pregnancy and medication during labour and delivery: Methodological considerations, in *Newborns and Parents*, (ed. V.L. Smeriglio), Lawrence Erlbaum Associates, New Jersey.

FURTHER READING

Bower, T.G.R. (1985) *The Perceptual World of the Child*, 2nd edn, Fontana, London.

This book offers a clear and interesting account of perceptual development which would be a useful next step to follow on from this chapter. It includes material concerning children with visual and auditory disabilities as well as many more examples of experiments revealing infant capacities.

Bower, T. (1989) *The Rational Infant: Learning in Infancy*, W.H. Freeman, New York.

Crawford, D. and Morris, M. (1994) *Neonatal Nursing*, Chapman and Hall, London.

This book provides an up to date account of neonatal nursing including some excellent work on, for example, play and the neonate and the care of the growing numbers of oxygen dependent infants.

Kelnar, C.J.H., Harvey, D. and Simpson, C. (1995) *The Sick Newborn Baby*, 3rd edn, Baillière Tindall, London.
The latest edition of this excellent book provides good accounts of the psychological care in relation to sick infants, particularly those requiring neonatal intensive care.

CHILDREN, FRIENDS AND FAMILIES 3

We have read in Chapter 2 how infants seem to be naturally inclined to be sociable and form relationships. Looking at the research in this area, one might be led to think that only mothers, or mothers and fathers, are important, yet normal infants and children develop relationships with other adults, and with other children (Rutter, 1995). In fact, interaction with peers (children of a similar age) is considered so important that Carlson (1984) is moved to suggest that 'interaction with peers is probably the most important factor in social development'. Why do children seem to need other children? How do relationships between children begin and develop? What kinds of relationships do brothers and sisters have with each other? What is the relevance of such information to dealing with children while they are in hospital? These questions are of particular relevance to those caring for children.

CHILDREN AND FRIENDS

Schaffer and Emerson (Schaffer, 1990) found, in their study of Glasgow children, that most infants formed attachments to several people, not just their mothers but also fathers, brothers, sisters, grandparents and neighbours. At 10 months of age, 41 per cent of the children had only one person to whom they were attached, yet by 18 months only 13 per cent were found to have just one attachment. It appears that it is not just the availability of a person, or the caretaking functions (dressing, washing, feeding) that attract babies to someone else; rather it is the sensitivity and responsiveness of other people to them.

Having more than one attachment appears to be an important part of social and emotional development. Research with monkeys by Harlow and his colleagues (Harlow and Harlow, 1969) has shown that contact with peers is essential to social development; infant monkeys that are raised only with their mothers, and have no opportunity to play with other young monkeys, do not develop normal social patterns of behaviour. When faced with other monkeys later on they either cower in fear, or are unusually aggressive. Their sexual responses are inappropriate and, if they do mate successfully, the female monkeys make poor mothers, tending to neglect or abuse their babies. Other studies from Harlow's laboratory (Novak and Harlow, 1975) have shown that the over-fearful response shown by a monkey reared in isolation from both mother and peers can later be eliminated by other young monkeys; if the isolated monkey is gradually brought into social situations by placing it first with a younger monkey, it gradually learns how to interact with older monkeys, in spite of its earlier deprivation.

A study by Fuhrman, Rahe and Hartup (cited in Carlson, 1984) used this 'juvenile therapist' technique with human children who were socially withdrawn, and found the young therapists were very successful. The children were aged between $2\frac{1}{2}$ and $6\frac{1}{2}$ years, and were socially withdrawn, spending very little time playing with peers. Each child was paired with another socially normal child for a series of ten play sessions of 20 minutes each. Interestingly, the children who were paired with *younger* 'therapists' showed the most improvement, although all were noticeably more sociable. It may be that a younger child is seen as less threatening, giving the older one more confidence to make friends.

Other studies with human children suggest that peer interaction is crucially important to development, and even more so when normal warm relationships with adults are not available. One particularly sad example was documented by Freud and Dann (1951). They studied six German Jewish children whose parents were murdered during World War II. During their first year the orphans were placed together in a small nursery in a concentration camp and then brought to England after the war. At first they were very hostile towards their adult caretakers, and it became clear that amongst all the tragedy, fear and rejection in the concentration camp they had developed extremely strong attachments to each other. They showed an amazing degree of tenderness and caring towards each other, and became very upset when separated, even if only for a few minutes. No child would go upstairs or go for a walk without the others. Eventually, they did develop affection for the adults who cared for them, but the intense nature of their relationships with each other shows how young children can, and indeed do, become extremely attached to persons other than parents.

There is other research showing that such friendships can and do occur very early on in life. Rubin (1980) cites a study by Lee in 1973, where a group of infants aged between 8 and 10 months were observed in their day-care centre. One of the babies, Jenny, was more consistently approached than were other members of the group, and one, Patrick, was more consistently avoided. Jenny was a responsive, lively child who seldom terminated social contacts that had been initiated by others. Patrick, on the other hand, was a belligerent and unfriendly baby, who frequently grabbed others and was reluctant to end encounters that he had initiated. But when others initiated contacts with him, he was passive and unresponsive. Patrick did not smile, laugh or otherwise display positive feelings on a single one of the occasions in which he was contacted by another baby. To put it bluntly, Patrick was no fun whereas Jenny had clearly learned the art of making friends very early on. It is likely that Patrick needed friends, but he did not now how to behave in a way that other babies found rewarding. Children like Patrick may benefit from some encouragement in this area since friendship serves particular functions for children.

Hay (1994) discusses evidence that children of 2 years of age or earlier show another type of social behaviour not usually associated with youngsters, that of altruism. They will offer help and comfort to another child who is hurt, at least occasionally. An interesting point in the research in this field is that children are more likely to do this if they are encouraged to be more helpful generally, and are given genuinely responsible tasks.

WHAT IS THE FUNCTION OF FRIENDSHIP?

It appears from the various studies that there are four main ways in which children serve distinct functions for one another through their friendships. Firstly, relationships with other children provide opportunities for learning particular social skills which are not normally learnt in child–parent relationships. Rubin (1980) points out that parents often make communication too easy for their own children, whereas friends do not allow this luxury. Social skills are very important in life, and children need to experience relationships which make varying kinds of demands on them. Children may, for example, find that their parents give in to their every wish, or they may have been taught to be totally malleable, doing whatever others tell them, or they may expect to be praised for everything they do. Children reinforce some behaviours in their friends by attention or approval, and punish others. The way other children respond is an important modifying influence and there is need for an honest peer group to teach children the subtleties of social interaction. Also, in pretend games with others, patterns of social behaviour are worked out and practised, and children learn about rules and their own strengths or weaknesses relative to their peers. Dunn (1996) writes on this point that children are interested in what others think of them and about how they are viewed by their peers.

This brings us to the second function of peer relationships: friendships give children an opportunity to compare themselves in a meaningful way with others, so that they can acquire some notion of 'self'. We only know what we are like by what people tell us, and by comparing our own performances with those of others. Adults are so very different from children in most aspects of behaviour that they do not serve a useful function as comparison points for children. Rutherford (1997) suggests that it is the perception of similarity that lies at the heart of babies' and children's attraction to their peers, in much the same way that older children and adults are most likely to be attracted to those who have similar interests and views to their own (Baron and Byrne, 1984). Rubin (1980) also notes that even young babies distinguish clearly between peers and adults, and tend to act more positively to unfamiliar peers than to unfamiliar adults.

It is this similarity that lies at the root of the third main function of friendship for children. Peers very often like similar things, such as saying the same silly phrase *ad infinitum* (or *ad nauseam*) which would become extremely tedious to adults. Friends will do the sorts of activities that would try the patience of most adults, simply because they are at the same stage of development, and therefore enjoy doing the same things over and over again. However much adults try to appear engrossed in the game, children may sense that their heart is not always in it, that they are just being humoured. Rubin (1980, p. 72) notes however that in both children's and adults' friendships, similarity is only a part of the attraction.

> *Most friendships also depend on complementarity – a fit between two people in which each brings something distinctive to the relationship and in which, as a result, each can learn something from the other.*

A fourth function of childhood friendships is that they satisfy a strong early developing need for a sense of belonging. Fine (1985) discusses that particular types of relationship can be seen in adults. There is an emotional security from a single close relationship with husband/wife, boyfriend/girlfriend, and there is a sense of community that comes from relationships with friends, neighbours and colleagues. These types of relationship are separate and cannot substitute for each other, a network of friends cannot compensate for the loss of a close relation through death or desertion, and also the presence of a single emotional attachment cannot alleviate the loneliness most people experience without friends and colleagues (at least, after the initial, engrossing interest has worn off). Evidence reviewed by Dunn (1996) suggests that this specialization of children's relationships begins early in life, with parents on the one hand and children on the other.

It is clear that children fulfil important functions for each other as they develop. Of course, there are individual differences in children's needs for other people, just as there are in adults. Many children have a need for moments of privacy and solitude. We also need to realize that children's friendships, again like adults', have destructive as well as constructive elements. 'Special' pairs of friends can reject others ('Go away, we don't want you with us') or stereotype them ('There's Jason, he's thick'). There can be jealousy and resentment and cruelty. Again, however, this merely serves to emphasize the major function of friendship in teaching about social interaction; all the above features are present in adult relationships, and need to be encountered in childhood so that children can practise dealing with them.

THE NATURE AND DEVELOPMENT OF CHILDREN'S FRIENDSHIPS

In the earliest stages of friendship, infants explore other infants in the same way they would explore a toy – poking, twisting, pulling and biting, interspersed with retreats back to their mother or father. The beginnings of identifiable social interaction with peers come towards the end of the first year, when friends are distinguished from inanimate objects because they can initiate and respond to social behaviours. They offer objects, they smile. In fact, offered toys often serve as the launching point for friendships by providing a common focus of attention, much like talk of the weather for adults. Toys require children to coordinate their behaviour so that they can make use of the toys. Without toys there is still interaction, but of a different kind with more touching, smiling and gesturing, and more copying of each other's actions (Foster *et al.*, 1989).

By $2\frac{1}{2}$ years of age, friendships contain all the basic features of adult social interaction: sustained attention, turn-taking and mutual responsiveness. However, up to about 5 years, friends are seen by children as 'momentary physical playmates' (Rubin, 1980). Friendships may endure, but equally may be transient. Young children are very definite about friendship, they do not yet understand that one can regard another person both positively and negatively at the same time. This seems to be related to their immature powers of reasoning, which makes them likely to deal with negative feelings about another child by deciding that they are not friends any more ('I'm not your friend, you can't come to my party').

Also, young children do not make friends in the same way as older children and adults, partly because they tend to be totally blunt. Verbal means of entry into a group often do not work. 'Hello, what are you doing? Can I play?' is likely to be remarkably unsuccessful in a pre-school group; 'Hello' is ignored, 'What are you doing' greeted with 'We're making a castle and you're not' and 'Can I play?' is met with 'No'. Children learn this early on, and develop a strategy of hovering around the players until they see a suitable entry point, usually in terms of activity rather than words. Children actually begin their friendships in a different way from the way adults enter into a relationship. It is considered rude if an adult begins a conversation by talking about him or herself, yet Rubin (1980) notes that children nearly always do this, with phrases like 'I've got jelly for my tea', or 'My teddy's got a headache'.

Early friendships show little evidence of sex preferences, but by the age of 11 years, sex segregation is almost total. Work by Fine (1980) suggests that the topic of conversation important among friends (e.g. sex and aggression in male pre-adolescent groups) precludes mixed sex friendships, as well as being unsuitable for adult–child interaction. Another likely contributing factor is that children within our culture are encouraged to divide according to sex from an early age, for example in sports and class activities. With regard to research in this area, it is worth pointing out that often the differences between the sexes attract more interest and tend to be published in research journals, but studies which fail to find differences may not be so readily published. This can give a biased impression by making one think that all the research does is discover differences.

Is play important?

Greig (1997) discusses the question of whether play is important in her excellent introduction to play theories. She points out that each stage of development is accompanied by a different kind of play, from the early learning and exploring of the infant to the complete rule-governed games of the 11-year-old. As children play, they are not only taking in information about their world, but also discovering the cause and effect of interactions with other people. They learn about the language and customs of their own society by watching others and then practising in play. Children under about 3 years of age tend to specialize in what is often called 'parallel play', where two or three children may be using the same objects or toys, but each plays independently. Later, around 3 to 4 years of age, we more 'cooperative play' where two or three children play together towards a common aim (e.g. building a toy house, or putting a toy together).

The friendships evident in play sessions between under-5s appear to be based on proximity and shared interests, and are not necessarily lasting relationships. Friends are people who are available, who will be there to play with you. Children aged between 5 and 12 years, however, are more likely to have stable positive friendships that play important roles in their lives. Children older than 11 or 12 years put much more emphasis on the psychological attributes of friendship, intimate and mutual sharing, a relationship which takes place over a period of time (Graham and Rutter, 1985). Taylor and Müller (1995, p. 37) cite a 13-year-old girl:

> *Friends are great to shop with and have a laugh with. They help you with stuff and give you truthful answers. You can tell them things and share things with them, share secrets. ... You love friends in a 'friend' way...*

When looking at play, it should of course be remembered that not everything young children do together is play. They also fight and argue, or just watch each other, and learn a great deal about social interaction from 'non-play' activities. It is also interesting to note that young children will differ in their play activities depending upon who their play partner is (e.g. close friends, sibling, mother) which clearly has implications for nurses. Dunn (1996), for example, suggests that ability to manage conflict in play situations will differ according to the context of the particular interaction.

CROSS-AGE FRIENDSHIPS

As well as sex-segregation in our society, age-segregation is widely practised, particularly in school where teachers may argue that the intellectual and social goals of education are best achieved if all the children in one group are at the same level of maturity. It is not only teachers who influence this. Rubin (1980), who includes in his book a chapter devoted entirely to cross-age friendships, points out that when parents move to a new area, they often make sure that there are other children of the same age, so that their sons and daughters can 'make friends'. From evidence cited by Rubin, it is clear that children in mixed age groups remain likely to establish their closest ties with children their own age, and it is unlikely that mixed age friendships can substitute for same-age friendships. But children can gain additional benefit from others older or younger than themselves. Competitiveness is reduced, younger children gain the stimulation of a relationship with someone who is more able than they are, yet close enough to understand their difficulties, and older children gain a sense of pride, achievement and responsibility in helping younger ones. Leiderman (1989) suggests that in societies in which cross-age interaction is the norm, children become less dependent and demanding with their parents and learn social behaviours which last throughout their lives from an 'older, larger, stronger and more competent member of his or her peer group'.

The most prevalent example of cross-age interaction that we have in our society is that between brothers and sisters, and it is to these relationships that we now turn. With the exception of work by Judy Dunn and her colleagues (Dunn and Kendrick, 1982; Dunn, 1984; Dunn, 1996) this is an area which attracted little interest in the past, which is perhaps surprising, considering the difference the presence of a sibling makes in family life. Boer and Dunn (1992) have edited a useful book on the subject of sibling relationships which contains a wealth of work in the field of cross-age interaction between siblings. Work in this field clearly raises questions about 'only children' which has recently been the focus of some interest by researchers (Richards and Goodman, 1996) as well as children born following *in vitro* fertilization, who are often only children (van Balen, 1996; Colpin *et al.*, 1995). Work has also been carried out which looks at how 'only' children experience the birth of a sibling. An earlier detailed study of sibling relationships (Dunn and Kendrick, 1982) expresses clearly (p. 1) the impact of another child in the family:

> *With the birth of a sibling, the world of a firstborn child is transformed. Never again will mother be alone ... 'Why have you ruined my life?' a precocious 4-year-old asked his mother when his brother was born.*

The data from this project are discussed more fully in a text by Dunn (1984), entitled simply *Sisters and Brothers*.

The 4-year-old child quoted above gives one view of siblings, yet children very often take great interest in their younger siblings, and the younger ones gain from having older ones in terms of help and entertainment. The view of conflict between siblings is perhaps the more usual perception. Mussen *et al.* (1990) suggest that, although in some cases brothers and sisters are very close, in far more cases the relationships are characterized by hostility.

Rubin (1980) suggests that age-segregation outside the family is the main reason for the frequent failure of siblings to become friends. In terms of social skills, the rough and tumble of sibling relationships must be good preparation for outside relationships, even if this is not appreciated by the siblings themselves.

SIBLINGS' REACTIONS TO ILLNESS

Of particular relevance are those studies that have looked at the effect on children when one of their brothers or sisters is ill and/or hospitalized. Harris (1979) asked children due to go into hospital what they would wish for if they could have only 3 wishes, and a number of the replies related to brothers and sisters. A 7-year-old said 'I wish my sister wasn't born' and an 11-year-old said 'I'd like a flat for me and my sister' (p. 234). In hospital, however, the first child missed his younger sister, and looked forward eagerly to her visits. The second child had a row with his sister the day before hospitalization and had nothing good to say about her throughout his stay.

Gath (1989), looking at families of chronically ill children, found problem behaviour and academic difficulties in siblings. Black (1994) also reports on studies which have found a two-fold increase in emotional disorders in siblings of children with life-threatening illness. Sloper and While (1996) found similar negative behavioural changes in a study of the siblings of children with cancer. On the other hand Stewart *et al.* (1992) found no significant negative impact on healthy children with an ill sibling, although in some siblings there was evidence of marked levels of distress. Stewart *et al.* stressed however that there were significant effects on family life which is an important factor in determining how a sibling reacts. Given that some siblings do develop behavioural changes that are worrisome and may render them more vulnerable to stress, and since these affect the family's ability to cope generally, the health care team is required to provide intervention and support. Taylor (1980) provides some useful guidance. For example (under the heading 'Who needs intervention?') she notes that children undergoing stresses of their own (such as starting school or moving house) will be particularly at risk during a sibling's illness, as will those who had poor relationships with their parents prior to the sick child's illness, and those who have not yet developed coping strategies to deal with new life experiences. Taylor also emphasizes that certain conditions in the ill child may make a well child more likely to suffer. These include mental retardation, multiple handicaps, other chronic disorders such as diabetes or cystic fibrosis, conditions which involve alteration of body image such as burns or massive trauma, and terminal illness. All these will have already involved the well child in disruption of routine. The types of sibling behaviour to watch out for include the development of physical symptoms (e.g. gastrointestinal problems, headaches or other vague pains, and symptoms imitating aspects of the ill child's condition), change in academic performance or attendance, changes in mood and social behaviour (e.g. irritability, withdrawal from friends, overt jealousy, being excessively demanding and bullying), regressive behaviours (e.g. enuresis, thumbsucking and clinging) and lastly anxiety-related habits (e.g. nightmares, nailbiting, stuttering or increased fearfulness).

Taylor's suggestions for nursing intervention begin with the provision of information to siblings, mainly to reduce the likelihood of siblings making up explanations which may be more frightening than fact. Siblings also need to know how the illness will affect them. Adolescents and older school-aged children may, for instance, be concerned about any genetic or epidemiological factors that are relevant to them: 'Specifically, they want to know if they are likely to develop the illness themselves or pass it on to their offspring' (Taylor, 1980). The next stage of intervention is support in adjusting to the illness and, lastly, referral if necessary. As Taylor notes, 'child psychologists or psychiatrists, social workers or school personnel are resources for supplementing the nurse's interactions with the family' and, when given encouragement, parents may openly share their concerns about their well children. The parent who appears to be coping very well, then suddenly seems to be unable to manage, may be finding things rather difficult at home.

FRIENDS IN HOSPITAL

Looking at the effect of other children in a ward environment, Pill (cited in Stacey *et al.*, 1970) found that children seemed less likely to give support to their fellows in distress than adults would in a similar situation. Out of 284 recorded instances of crying, a child intervened in only 30 cases; in fact they were more likely to mock or tease. However, responding to crying is a narrow view of a relationship, and it is possible to successfully enlist the help of older children with younger ones in hospital, both to give the younger child the kind of informed personalized relationship that he or she would have at home from a sibling, and to give the older child a rewarding interest and the warm response of a smaller child's affection. It is clear that children do respond to the distress of other children. Comments from the children in Harris's (1979) study about other, usually younger children, were frequent in answer to the question 'What didn't you like about the hospital?':

> ... *seeing the ill and unhappy babies (12 year old);*
> ... *the nurses telling the little ones who were crying not to be a baby (6 year old);*
> ... *nurses shouting at the little ones (6 year old);*
> ... *I felt sorry for the babies who cried for their mums (7 year old);*
> ... *hearing small children cry depressed me (12 year old).*

Comments such as these led a number of the parents in this study to suggest the separation of both ill and not-so-ill and older and younger children. For example one mother of a 6 year old made the following comment (p. 177):

> *Babies and younger children should be separated from older children as their crying for 'Mummy' upset the older ones, and it seemed to them that the nurses were just ignoring their cries.*

Children do not understand about staff shortages, or the other reasons why babies may be left crying, and see it as neglect. Separation of age groups may help, but this would mean that the younger children would not benefit from the support of the older ones. Harris found that older children were often a comfort to the younger ones; one 10 year old was asked by a nurse to try and cheer up a younger crying child. He said, 'Yes, I don't mind making myself useful', and within a short time the younger child was chuckling with delight, although previous attempts by adults on the ward had not been successful. If age groups were segregated, other arrangements (such as a programme of 'visiting' between wards) would need to be made to keep open this avenue of support.

In general, Harris found that the presence of other children was very rewarding for the children in her sample, enjoyed at the time of stay and remembered with pleasure afterwards. Friendships were quickly made, and the discharge of a new-found friend was the only cause of crying in eight of the children. Those children who were cheerful throughout their short stay in hospital were the ones who had made the most friends and conversely those who were upset were the children who made no friends. It is not possible to distinguish cause and effect here however, since the unhappy children were in no frame of mind to strike up new friendships.

The age group admitted with the children appeared to be important; when three or four of the same age group were admitted together, the children were more likely to be cheerful than when four of a wide age range came into the ward at one time. Staff were aware of this, and attempts were made to arrange admission so that similar aged children arrived together, but this was not always possible where waiting lists had to be respected.

Very often the children played, talked and collaborated in pranks together. One group always pretended to be asleep during the doctors' rounds, then got up with a sigh of relief after they had gone. Another group chose to play football one evening when there was nothing on television, and the ball broke a window in the ward, via a lampshade. None of the children would say who did the kicking, and the researcher was silenced with warning looks. There were often competitions to see who could keep sweets in their lockers before the nurses discovered the hidden booty. The children complained to each other too. One 9 year old was heard to say to another at dinner time 'I think I'll have to have another cut in my tummy to get these beefburgers out', and a 12 year old announced 'There's more people than chips at this table'.

Peterson (1989) comments on the communication system that can develop between children in hospital with the younger ones exploring their uncertainties together in play. Older children tend to exchange more direct information about their illnesses and treatment. Patient culture, for many children and adolescents, is a primary source of anxiety reduction.

Friends outside the hospital were also very important to the children in Harris's (1979) study. They were generally interested and supportive; many of the children received letters from or were visited by friends while they were in hospital, which seemed to help them to maintain links with their normal lives for the short time during which they would otherwise have been cut off from them. It is likely that for children hospitalized for a longer period, this would be particularly crucial.

Apart from children who are hospitalized for long periods, there are also particular forms of treatment which may necessitate special consideration of children's needs for other children. Some treatment, such as intensive care or barrier nursing, will preclude the presence of other children; in such cases, encouraging parents to bring in cards or perhaps tape recordings from the child's friends can be beneficial and will be much appreciated. Enforced immobility is often particularly traumatic for children, but is made even more so by the limitations it sets on social interaction. Where children cannot go off and find friends (for example in a wheelchair or on a stretcher), it is important to ensure that other children can come and talk to them.

A further consideration in any discussion about children being visited by other children must be the effect on staff. There may be sound medical reasons why visits by other children may not be advisable, such as the possibility of infection, but it is obvious that visiting should only be restricted when there is really a good reason to do so, and not merely for the sake of administrative convenience. It is a simple matter for a nurse to keep an eye on visited children to ensure that they are not becoming tired or excited in a way that might set back their recovery. If they are, then this can be gently explained to the visitors, who can be asked to come back later, after the child has had a little rest. When the visitors are children, it is in the interests of both the sick child and the visiting children that the visit should not be lengthy. Just long enough to keep the ill child in touch is often all that is required.

This section on the importance of friends to children in hospital is best summed up by a parent on p. 175 of Harris's (1979) study. She was one of the many mothers who commented on the value to their children of other children on the ward, and was answering the question 'What would you tell other parents whose child was due to come into hospital?'

Try and introduce your child formally to another child, so that he knows by name at least one person he can approach when parents and friends are not present.

Finally, it is worth noting that, until recently, there has been very little systematic investigation of the function and nature of children's friendships with other children. This seems surprising considering how interesting this area of child development is. Rubin (1980) suggests two possible reasons for this lack of research interest in children's friendships. Firstly, early theory led to an almost complete emphasis on the mother–child relationship, to the exclusion of research into a child's relationship with anyone else. Secondly, the lack of interest may have been a reflection of our society, where pre-school children had few formal opportunities (in the form of playgroups and nursery schools) to interact with other children of a similar age, or to be observed in such interactions. Mannarino (1980) adds that another reason for lack of systematic work in this area is that it is very difficult to look at all the many aspects of friendship within a research framework. He emphasizes that the research in this area is, even now, fragmented and often not related to any clear background theory (see also Buhrmester, 1992).

In spite of these problems, it is hoped that the account presented here will be enough to demonstrate that friends do appear to serve important functions to developing children. Siblings are important too, and we should respect the social needs of children, their siblings and friends; fulfilment of these needs appears to be an essential requirement for normal child development.

In practice ➤

- Friends serve central functions for children that parents do not, and so, in addition to making parents welcome in hospital, friends should also be encouraged, wherever the conditions for nursing care allow this. Peer relationships are particularly important when normal warm relationships with adults are not available.
- Children make friends in a different way from adults. Nurses may find it easier to get on with children if they get down to their (physical) level, and then say something about themselves, since this is the way children very often begin a relationship (e.g. 'I've got a little boy who is nearly as big as you'; 'I've got a funny name, do you want to know what it is?').
- If a child patient has siblings, it may be helpful to tell parents that brothers and sisters adjust better if they have only minor changes to their routine, such as spending more or less time with one or the other parent. The needs of the well children are still there, even though the child in hospital has the greatest need for the moment.
- The 'patient culture' is as important to children (even young ones) as it is to adults, and it is worth spending some time in thinking how it might best be encouraged and maintained in your ward. A room in which to talk and relax, or watch television with new friends and visitors will enable peers to support each other and to keep some continuity with home life.
- Children can benefit greatly from mixing with children older or younger than themselves, a situation they are almost certain to find in hospital. Older children can help and comfort younger ones, at the same time gaining a sense of pride, achievement and responsibility. This can be particularly meaningful for them in hospital, where they can feel very helpless and vulnerable.

Baron, R.A. and Byrne, D. (1984) *Social Psychology: Understanding Human Interaction*, 4th edn, Allyn and Bacon, Boston, Mass.

Black, D. (1994) Terminal Illness and Bereavement, in *Child and Adolescent Psychiatry: Modern Approaches*, 3rd edn, (eds M. Rutter, E. Taylor and L. Hersov), Blackwell, Oxford.

Boer, F. and Dunn, J. (eds) (1992) *Children's Sibling Relationships: Development and Clinical Issues*, Erlbaum Associates, Hillsdale, New Jersey.

Buhrmester, D. (1992) The Developmental Courses of Sibling and Peer Relationships, in *Children's Sibling Relationships: Development and Clinical Issues*, (eds F. Boer and J. Dunn), Erlbaum Associates, Hillsdale, New Jersey.

Carlson, N.R. (1984) *Psychology: The Science of Behaviour*, Allyn and Bacon, Boston, Mass.

Colpin, H., Demyttenaere, K. and Vandemeulebroecke, L. (1995) New Reproductive Technology and the Family: the parent-child relationship following *in vitro* fertilization. *Journal of Child Psychology and Psychiatry*, 36(8), 1429–42.

Dunn, J. (1984) *Sisters and Brothers*, Fontana, London.

Dunn, J. (1993) Young Children's Close Relationships: beyond attachment. *Individual Differences and Development Series*, vol. 4, Sage, Newbury Park.

Dunn, J. (1996) The Emanuel Miller Memorial Lecture 1995. Children's Relationships: bridging the divide between cognitive and social development. *Journal of Child Psychology and Psychiatry*, 37(5), 507–18.

Dunn, J. and Kendrick, C. (1982) *Siblings: Love, Envy and Understanding*, Grant McIntyre, London.

Fine, G.A. (1980) The natural history of pre-adolescent male friendship groups, in *Friendship and Social Relations in Children*, (eds H.C. Foot, A.J. Chapman and J.R. Smith), John Wiley, Chichester.

Fine, R. (1985) *The Meaning of Love in Human Experience*. John Wiley, New York.

Foster, R., Hunsberger, M. and Anderson, J. (1989) *Family Centred Nursing Care for Children*, W.B. Saunders, Philadelphia.

Freud, A. and Dann, S. (1951) An experiment in group upbringing, in *The Psychoanalytic Study of the Child: Volume VI*, International Universities Press, New York.

Gath, A. (1989) Living with a mentally handicapped brother or sister. *Archives of Disease in Childhood*, 64, 513–6.

Graham, P. and Rutter, M. (1985) Adolescent disorders, in *Child and Adolescent Psychiatry*, (eds M. Rutter and L. Hersov), Blackwell Scientific Publications, Oxford.

Greig, A. (1997) Play, Language and Learning, in *Early Childhood Studies: an Holistic Introduction*, (eds J. Taylor and M. Woods), Arnold, London.

Harlow, H.F. and Harlow, M.K. (1969) Effects of Various Mother–Infant Relationships on Rhesus Monkey Behaviours, in *Determinants of Infant Behaviour*, (ed. B.M. Foss), Methuen, London.

Harris, P.J. (1979) *Children, their Parents and Hospital*, Unpublished PhD thesis, University of Nottingham.

Hay, D.F. (1994) Prosocial Development. *Journal of Child Psychology and Psychiatry*, 35(1), 29–71.

Leiderman, P.H. (1989) Relationship disturbances and development through the life cycle, in *Relationship Disturbances in Early Childhood*, (eds A.J. Sameroff and R.N. Emde), Basic Books, New York.

Mannarino, A.P. (1980) The development of children's friendships, in *Friendship and Social Relationships in Children*, (eds H.C. Foot, A.J. Chapman and J.R. Smith), John Wiley, Chichester.

Mussen, P.H., Conger, J.J., Kagan, J. and Huston, A.C. (1990) *Child Development and Personality*, 7th edn, Harper and Row, New York.

Novak, M.A. and Harlow, H.F. (1975) Social rehabilitation of isolate-reared monkeys. *Developmental Psychology*, 6, 487–96.

Peterson, G. (1989) Let the children play. *Nursing*, Series 3(4), 22–5.

Richards, H. and Goodman, R. (1996) Are only children different? A study of child psychiatric referrals. A research note. *Journal of Child Psychology and Psychiatry*, 37(6), 753–8.

Rubin, Z. (1980) *Children's Friendships*, Fontana, London.

Rutherford, D. (1997) Children's Relationships, in *Early Childhood Studies: an Holistic Introduction*, (eds J. Taylor and M. Woods), Arnold, London.

Rutter, M. (1995) Clinical Implications of Attachment Concepts: Retrospect and Prospect. *Journal of Child Psychology and Psychiatry*, 36(4), 549–71.

Schaffer, H.R. (1990) *Making Decisions about Children*, Basil Blackwell, Oxford.

Sloper, P. and While, D. (1996) Risk factors in the Adjustment of Siblings of Children with Cancer. *Journal of Child Psychology and Psychiatry*, 37(5), 597–607.

Stacey, M., Dearden, R., Pill, R. and Robinson, D. (1970) *Hospitals, Children and their Families*, Routledge and Kegan Paul, London.

Stewart, D.A., Stein, A., Forrest, G.C. and Clark, D.M. (1992) Psychological Adjustment in Siblings of Children with Chronic Life Threatening Illness. *Journal of Child Psychology and Psychiatry*, 33(4), 779–84.

Taylor, S.C. (1980) Siblings need a plan of care too. *Pediatric Nursing*, 6, 9–13.

Taylor, J. and Müller, D. (1995) *Nursing Adolescents: Research and Psychological Perspectives*, Blackwell Science, Oxford.

van Balen, F. (1996) Child-rearing following *in vitro* fertilization. *Journal of Child Psychology and Psychiatry*, 37(6), 687–94.

FURTHER READING

Boer, F. and Dunn, J. (eds) (1992) *Children's Sibling Relationships: Development and Clinical Issues*, Erlbaum Associates, Hillsdale, New Jersey.
An excellent collection of papers relating to sibling relationships. It includes work undertaken with disabled siblings.

Dunn, J. (1984) *Sisters and Brothers*, Fontana, London.
A very readable account of sibling relationships. Includes both discussion of research and practical guidelines for parents and health professionals. Highly recommended.

Greig, A. (1997) Play, Language and Learning, in *Early Childhood Studies: an Holistic Introduction*, (eds J. Taylor and M. Woods), Arnold, London.
This chapter is exceptionally well presented and provides an excellent introduction to relevant theories.

THE DEVELOPMENT OF CHILDREN'S UNDERSTANDING

4

In Chapters 2 and 3 we have built up a picture of the development of children, with the main emphasis being on relationships with other people. In this chapter, the emphasis is wider so as to explore the way children understand events in the world around them. The discussion centres around how a child's view of illness and hospitalization will be affected by his or her stage of cognitive development which, put simply, is the development of the ability to reason and think.

JEAN PIAGET

There are a number of approaches to cognitive development, and all agree that there are important differences between the cognitive processing of children and that of adults (Greig, 1997). The most comprehensive and widely referred to work on children's cognitive development is that of the Swiss scientist Jean Piaget (1896–1980), who began his interest in children's thinking when he looked at the incorrect answers children gave to a number of interesting problems. His lifetime's work was devoted to the investigation of cognitive processes in children, which he called *schemas*.

Piaget first questioned many children between the ages of 3 and 12 years to discover how they saw the things in their world. He was not interested in differences between children, rather in finding the similar and systematic ways of reasoning and thinking characteristic of children of roughly equivalent ages. He found that at different times during development children appeared to be capable of different kinds of understanding. He described these in the form of a series of stages. It is important for the health professional to have an awareness of the typical characteristics of thinking at each stage, as children's understanding of illness and hospitalization is limited by their stage of general cognitive development.

STAGES OF COGNITIVE DEVELOPMENT

When reading through the brief outline of the four major stages given below, it is important to remember that above all Piaget emphasized the contribution of the child in interacting with the environment to construct his or her understanding. The child's knowledge or understanding at any one time is based neither wholly on experience, nor wholly on existing schemas, but on an interaction between the two. You may find it useful to speculate, as you read through the description of stages, on how illness and hospitalization might be viewed by a child at different stages.

The sensori–motor stage

In this first stage (approximate age range 0–2 years), babies are discovering the relationship between what they do and the consequences of what they do. It is called the sensori–motor stage because learning is mainly through the senses and physical activity. Babies learn how far they have to stretch their arm to grasp a rattle, what happens when they push their plate of casserole to (and over) the edge of the highchair tray, what happens when rattles are shaken, dropped, banged and chewed. At first, objects only appear to exist in terms of what a baby can do to them. If a cloth is placed over a toy for which a 7 month old is reaching, the baby appears to lose all interest, as if the toy no longer existed. A 1 year old will look actively for the toy, even though it is out of sight. In Piaget's terms, the baby has attained the concept of *object permanence*. This is important, since it means that 1 year olds know, for example, that their mother still exists even though she is not in sight; they are therefore much more likely to cry for her than are younger babies.

During the first year babies change in their attitude towards objects. At first, objects are simply things to act upon (can I suck it? can I hit it?), whereas towards the end of the first year the object is examined as though it presents an interesting problem to the baby, as if there is an attempt to understand as the object is looked at, felt, explored, turned around and around. In Piaget's terms the baby has a mental schema for the object and can compare each new object or event with the schema already acquired from earlier experience. Adults can make judgements about objects and events very quickly because they have had years of experience in dealing with them, but for a baby the process is lengthy. The knowledge is acquired through action; there is a story that a famous athlete once tried to imitate an 18 month old baby's every move and after four hours he collapsed with exhaustion. Restriction of movement at this stage is therefore potentially harmful. It is important that babies should be able to explore their environment safely.

The pre-operational (or pre-logical) stage

Children at this stage (approximate age range 2–7 years) are prone to invest many objects with life (animism) and to give them their own personal identities. This tendency can be used by nurses to obtain cooperation. Beales (1983), for example, suggests that the nurse should not talk about 'a bad knee' but 'an unhappy knee', and the child is responsible for keeping it happy; 'Mr Arm' may not like the injection, but should put up with a bit of nastiness to ensure unhappy 'Mr Knee' gets a magic potion. Beales' suggestions reflect another important development; by the age of 2 years most children have begun to use language where words symbolize or represent things and events in their world. Objects are also used symbolically; a piece of wood can stand for a boat, a chair can represent a horse. However, in spite of this sophistication, there are many rules (or, in Piaget's terms, operations) which are not yet available to the child. For example, as adults we can 'conserve', that is we know that the weight of a substance is not altered when its shape is changed, we know that liquids do not change in volume when they are poured from a small container into a larger container, we know that two rows of six sweets will still each contain six sweets, even if those in one row are squashed up together. Children in the pre-operational (or pre-logical) stage cannot think reliably in the logical way that adults take for granted.

Piaget demonstrated this through his conservation experiments, all of which had the following essential principles in common (Atkinson *et al.*, 1996, p. 62).

1. The objects are presented to the child so that they look the same length, weight, number or volume (two identical glasses are filled with the same amount of water, two balls of clay have the same weight, or two rows of six buttons are the same length, as in Figure 4.1).
2. The child is asked whether the two objects or sets of objects are the same and, if necessary, adjustments are made until the child accepts that they are the same.
3. A change is made which makes the objects look different, although the actual length, number, weight, etc., is unaffected (e.g. water from one glass is poured into a taller, thinner glass, one of the balls of clay is rolled into a sausage shape, one of the rows of buttons is spread out so that the length of the row is greater, as in Figure 4.2).
4. The child is asked again whether the two objects or sets of objects are the same.

If on second questioning, the child maintains that the objects are still the same, even though they no longer look the same, then he or she is said

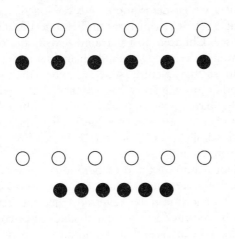

Figure 4.1

The classic conservation experiment, Stage I. Two rows of six buttons are put in front of the child so that they look the same number. The child agrees that there is the same number of white as black, and getting this agreement constitutes Stage II.

Figure 4.2

The classic conservation experiment, Stage III. One of the rows of buttons is spread out so that the length of the row is greater. In Stage IV, the child is asked whether there are the same number of buttons in the white row as the black row. Children under 7 years commonly say that there are more white buttons than black.

to conserve length, or weight or whatever the attribute may be. Otherwise the child is said to fail to conserve, or to be a nonconserver.

Children under the age of 7 years commonly fail to conserve. For example a 4 year old, if asked to make a judgement about amount, will agree that two balls of clay are the same but when one ball is rolled into a sausage shape will say it has more (or less) clay. One reason for this, according to Piaget, is that children under 6 or 7 years will tend to focus or centre on just one aspect of the shape. If they say the sausage is bigger they are centring on the length; if smaller they are centring on the width. So, children's thinking during this stage is very much dominated by visual impressions. Turner (1984, p. 45) sums up this stage of development very aptly when she writes:

> *Pre-operational children, sensibly enough, start from where they are, and to a greater or lesser extent distort reality as they attempt to assimilate it, or make sense of it, using the cognitive schemes, or ways of understanding, which they have developed.*

One consequence of this is that the child's thinking is centred on the self (egocentric) to a greater extent than it is in adults. Piaget used the term 'egocentric' not in the usual sense of 'selfish', but rather to mean that the young child centres on his or her own point of view or perspective and does not realise that others have a different point of view. His most well-known experiment demonstrating egocentricity is the 'three mountains task'. For this, Piaget used a model of three mountains distinguished from one another by colour and various features such as snow on one, a red cross at the top of another and a house on the peak of the third. The model was placed on a table and the child sat on one side. Piaget then produced a doll, put the doll at a different position and asked the child what the doll could see. To avoid the difficulty of a verbal description, one version of the task asked the child to look at a set of ten pictures and choose the one showing what the doll could see. Children up to around 8 years old could not usually do this successfully, the younger children (below about 6 years) tended in fact to choose the picture showing what they themselves saw. Research by other investigators has confirmed that children under 8 years do indeed have great difficulty with the three mountains task, although a number of experiments have since shown that children's thinking is not wholly egocentric, but it is certainly true that young children start from where they are.

Another major feature of the pre-operational stage of cognitive development is a lack of reversibility. Young children do not appear to realize that a series of actions can be reversed, that the clay in the above example could be returned to its original state. They concentrate on the present moment. To conserve, they would have to perform the action of transforming the clay in their heads, reasoning as follows: 'The two balls were the same. One has been squashed and rolled into a sausage. But, it could be made into the same ball again. Therefore the amount has not changed'. Pre-operational children cannot do this, whereas during the next stage (i.e., the concrete operational stage), children master conservation.

The concrete operational stage

Children at this stage (approximate age range 7–12 years) are no longer tricked by appearances. They can form internal pictures of a series of actions and they are more able to see the relationships between things. More flexibility is apparent in their approach to life. Whereas a pre-operational child thinks in absolutes, things are either good or bad, right or wrong, hurt or do not hurt, a concrete operational child can see things relatively; things can hurt a little or a lot. Piaget used the term 'concrete' because although there is a change in children's thinking (less egocentric and more logical), the understanding is still in relation to absolute objects, not to objects, events or relationships they have not yet experienced.

The formal operational stage

The major development in this stage (approximately 12 years and over) is that children can now think beyond the concrete here and now and think abstractly. They can imagine or hypothesize about alternatives. Reasoning about objects, people or events can be done symbolically, that is without the need for the things or events to be present.

We have built up a picture of how children's thinking develops. The difference between children's and adults' thinking appears not to be confined to how much they know, but the way they know. It is only as children mature cognitively and have many and varied experiences with their environment that they come to think in the logical way that we, as adults, take for granted. Piaget emphasized that children do not act like sponges passively soaking up knowledge, but assimilate (take in) experience as far as it is relevant to them and can be understood by them. As they mature they make use of their experiences to change their way of dealing with the world. The younger the child, the less complex the schemas, and the more reality will be distorted to fit the schemas. Piaget's description of cognitive development is an intriguing, immensely clever, seductive description of the course of cognitive development. But is it right?

CRITICISMS OF PIAGET

Some of the major criticisms of Piaget's work have centred on the methods he used to collect his data. Several researchers (Atkinson *et al.*, 1996; Bryant, 1974) have claimed that Piaget made his tasks too difficult for children and have showed that pre-school children can think logically when the tasks are simplified. Donaldson (1986) describes an experiment devised by Hughes which was similar to Piaget's mountain task, but provided a context which meant more to children. In the simplest version two intersecting walls were placed to form a cross and

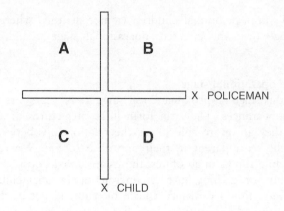

Figure 4.3

Experiment to demonstrate that children can see another person's point of view. If a boy doll is placed in Section A even young children know that the policeman cannot see him and that the boy can be seen by the policeman if placed in Section B.

two dolls were used representing a policeman and a little boy (see Figure 4.3). The policeman doll was placed where he could see the areas B and D, but A and C were hidden from his view by a wall. The child sat at the end of the wall between C and D. Hughes put the boy doll in A and asked the child if the policeman could see him there, then repeated the question for sections B, C and D in turn. Very few mistakes were made. Another policeman was then introduced and positioned as Figure 4.4. The child was told to hide the boy from both policemen, which of course required consideration of two different points of view. Hughes found that 90 per cent of under 5 year olds gave correct answers. It is likely that this was because Hughes' experiment made sense to them, they understood exactly what they were supposed to do. The motives and intentions of the characters are entirely comprehensible in such a context, as opposed to the abstract nature of the mountains task.

Similarly, in the conservation experiments, a major criticism is that the child is influenced by the situation in which an authoritative adult asks a question, accepts the answer, then changes something (rolls the ball of clay into a sausage shape). It is reasonable for a child to feel that the answer should be different the second time. In fact adults make this

Figure 4.4

Experiment to demonstrate that children can consider two different points of view. Even when the task is made more difficult by the introduction of another policeman, most under fives are successful.

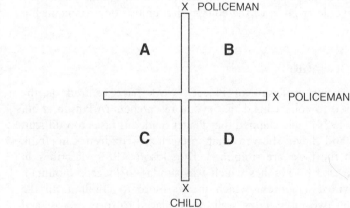

type of assumption in jokes like 'What do they call lemons in Los Angeles?' the answer is, of course, 'lemons', but most adults expect the answer to be different. In the conservation experiments, if a naughty teddy makes a change rather than a respected adult, children are more likely to give correct answers, showing that under some circumstances they can conserve. However, even with naughty teddy involved, many children still do not conserve, showing that their thinking is indeed different from that of adults. Many of these types of criticism relate to seeing the stages as steplike rather than continuous and sometimes overlapping. Piaget himself in his later work came round to seeing the stages in the latter way, in that a child may operate at one stage for one problem, and at another stage for a different problem.

Another criticism relates to the vagueness of Piaget's concepts. Schemas for example are rather abstract, and it is impossible to show they exist. Their presence can only be inferred from what children say and do. However, it may be extremely useful to be able to describe cognitive development in this way. It fits to some extent what evidence we have, and gives us a remarkably detailed source of guidance when we are attempting to explain things to children and understand what they are saying to us.

CHILDREN'S UNDERSTANDING OF ILLNESS AND HOSPITALIZATION

The large amount of research on Piaget's approach to child development confirms that understanding differs at various stages from early childhood to adulthood, and that it does so in a largely predictable fashion. Since illness, hospitalization and all that these entail are experiences encountered by many children, it seems likely that their understanding of these events will follow a similar progression. If this were so, detailed information about this progression would be of much value to the health professional who has to explain illness and events surrounding hospitalization to children. In recent years there has been growing awareness that patients' beliefs and assumptions about health and illness may have crucially important effects on compliance and recovery (Marteau, 1989). For children, in addition to the factors that affect comprehension in adults (Ley, 1988), the ability to understand information is further limited by their level of cognitive development and they are even more likely to distort the information available to them (Goodall, 1994). If we have the knowledge to predict the nature of the distortion this can provide guidelines to:

1. help improve explanations of illness and hospitalization;
2. provide sensitive reassurance for children;
3. gain greater understanding of what the child is saying to us;
4. gain some insight into how the child is interpreting all the strange occurrences that can accompany illness.

Does a child's understanding of illness change with age from egocentric notions such as 'I'm ill because I was naughty' to an increasing awareness of the many interacting factors causing disease? Is there a developing ability to think of events in hospital in relative terms rather than the absolute thinking enshrined in 'the nurse hurt me because she's horrible'? There has been an increasing amount of research addressing questions like these, and some useful answers are emerging.

Early research (Nagy, 1952) suggested that there were clear developmental changes in children's understanding of illness; it was not until after the age of 10 or 11 that children became aware of the interrelated factors in illness and treatment. It was left to later workers to investigate this in more detail. A number of researchers have interviewed normal healthy children to discover their understanding of the causes, prevention and treatment of illness (see for example, Bibace and Walsh, 1980; Perrin and Gerrity, 1981). Others have used drawings by children as a means of giving insight into cognitive and psychological functioning (Johnson, 1990). Millstein *et al.* (1981) talked specifically to adolescents, and a few studies have looked at the understanding of chronically ill children (Brewster, 1982; Beales, 1983; Bennett-Johnson, 1988). From all these studies it is clear that the child's understanding of illness does indeed parallel the understanding of other concepts such as conservation, although it appears to proceed more slowly. Although different researchers give different labels to the various stages they describe, the type of understanding of illness exhibited by children at each stage of development is remarkably consistent in all the research. By using the information available to us, we can build up a picture of the child's understanding of illness, hospitalization and treatment in the last three major stages formulated by Piaget, and discussed above. (The sensori–motor stage is not covered here since verbal explanations are inappropriate with such young children).

Pre-operational stage

Younger children at this stage (2 to 5 years old) see the cause of illness as external, concrete and remote from them, often doing its nasty work 'by magic' and certainly out of the child's control. They often conceive illness as being the outcome of their wrongdoing, and Brewster (1982) found that 5 and 6 year olds in her study routinely stated that medical procedures were done to punish them for being naughty. Because children at the pre-operational stage tend to focus on single aspects of experiences or objects without reference to the whole, they are unable to understand illness as a process, nor to have any conception of internal bodily mechanisms. The body is seen only in terms of its surface, the bit they can see. Important aspects of hospital to children are likely at this stage to be external, observable events (e.g. equipment, lights in the operating theatre, surface wounds, food, nurses' uniforms and strange beds) rather than a description of what is going on inside the body.

Later in this stage, perhaps related to their more sophisticated use of language, many children's responses to questions about illness have a stereotypical quality. They tend simply to repeat descriptions of the symptoms, actions or situations associated with the illness. Parental statements appear to be the main source. Illness, for example, is caused by going out without a coat in cold weather. From about the age of 5 years, there is some idea of the cause of illness being located in other people, although the nature of the link between the cause and the actual illness is not understood. Children at this stage think illness is caught. Perrin and Gerrity (1981) call this later pre-operational stage the 'contagion' period. However since there is no understanding of the mechanism of infection, children are likely to think that any illness can be caught. An interesting piece of nursing research by Norbeck (1981) suggests that children at this stage may find it difficult to recognize the same nurse who might have different facial expressions on two different occasions; they are unable to conserve facial identity. This suggestion requires further investigation, but may be important since children have little else to go on where uniforms are similar and their vision is restricted when they are, for example, lying down.

Concrete operational stage

The reasoning of the 6 to 8 years olds is more sophisticated, although they still see the cause of illness as exclusively external, but say that the agent must physically contact the child, or the child must physically engage in harmful activity. However there is still one physical cause for illness, usually germs, even in children with congenital heart disease (Brewster, 1982). The child can now link concrete symptoms to other bodily events, thus understanding the association between, for example, his or her rash, stomach ache and fever (Perrin and Gerrity, 1981; Swanwick, 1990). Later in this stage, although the ultimate cause of illness is seen as external, illness itself is seen as located inside the body and there is some notion of internalization of the agent by swallowing or inhaling. Yet even in this later stage, both cause and illness are described in only vague, nonspecific terms, showing confusion about internal organs and functions. The body is still equated almost entirely with its surface, and there is very little speculation by children under 10 years old as to what may be beneath the surface. Beales (1983) for example found that for children under 10 years of age with arthritis, feeling unwell was having a visibly red and swollen joint, although it is likely that children with chronic illness are ahead of their peers in their understanding (Goodall, 1994). An advantage of this view of illness is that, unlike an adult, a child will not be worried by thoughts of what might be going wrong inside the body. Children also begin to see the relationship between treatment and illness, and know that treatment is intended to help them get well again.

Formal operational stage

By this stage the cause of illness is described in terms of nonfunctioning or malfunctioning of an internal organ or process. There is an idea of the interaction between external cause and internal bodily response, such as infection and the body's lack of immunity, and an appreciation that there are many causes of illness. Later in this stage the child appreciates that a person's thoughts or feelings can affect the way the body functions, which shows an awareness of psychological factors.

Children now have the ability to imagine relationships and processes that they have not directly experienced. For example, in his work on juvenile arthritic patients, Beales (1983) stresses that children over 12 years of age show a growing concern about internal disease processes. The external signs of swelling and decreased mobility are now associated with internal damage and malfunction. Pain, instead of being just uncomfortable, will be more difficult to cope with since the child's level of cognitive development enables him or her to imagine the sinister implications of pain. A further result of being able to imagine things that have never been experienced can lead to a pessimistic view of the future for children with chronic illness. A younger child has no clear conception of adult life, whereas for an adolescent the realities can be foreseen and the limitations that illness may put on life be clearly imagined. Finally, where treatment is concerned, children can now infer empathy, they know that the nurse realizes the medical procedures are not necessarily pleasant.

FURTHER CONSIDERATIONS

To conclude this section on children's understanding of the meaning of illness and hospitalization, we should point out that at all stages there are other factors, apart from the level of cognitive development, that will play a part. The child's need for other people (Chapter 3) will influence the way that illness and hospitalization are seen. For example, Taylor and Müller (1995) suggest that adolescent peer company and contact with friends from outside hospital can be beneficial for both the ill adolescent and the friends. Both can have a more informed view of hospital and illness. This is particularly important when appearance is altered – it gives friends the chance to become accustomed to changed appearance and the ill adolescent more time to become accustomed to the reactions of others in a secure environment. Furthermore, children at every stage of cognitive development can feel the disruptions of friendship resulting from hospitalization and can benefit from visits and other contact with friends.

Another factor is that the ages given for the various stages are very approximate. For example, some 5 year olds are capable of understanding analogies (such as antibodies are like soldiers), whereas most will simply take the analogy completely literally. The most constructive starting point for any explanations, therefore, is the child; listen first to the child's own explanation. Jolly (1981a) suggests watching what children stare at in hospital and then asking what they think it is. Similarly, with medical procedures she suggests asking questions like 'How do you think they'll get the plaster off?', and 'How do you think your leg is under that plaster?', which gives an opportunity to confirm to an uncertain child that the leg is still there, even though it cannot be seen.

It is also the case that a child's understanding of explanations is influenced by the choice of words used. The words need to have only one possible meaning, or be very carefully explained. Pontious (1982) for example suggests avoiding the words 'cut' which implies pain, 'organs' which implies musical instruments, 'take' (temperature or blood pressure) which implies removal of something and 'test' which is not understood by under 5s, and denotes the possibility of pass or fail to the school-aged child. Jolly (1981b) tells the story of a little girl who was convinced her appendix consisted of Kleenex, because she heard it was made of tissues. She stresses that many of the words in common use in hospital (e.g. patella hammer, tube, sucker) can be very alarming. Goodall (1994) recounts a similar example of a little boy who became very worried when he thought the doctor had said he was going to fetch the 'deathoscope'. Although it is very important to talk in terms that a child at a particular cognitive stage will understand and be familiar with, the use of analogies must be carefully thought out. Beales (1983) gives an example of a young boy with a chest complaint who had not previously given a moment's thought to what might be going on inside him. He was far from reassured when the doctor explained that his lungs are like balloons; all the balloons he had known had had extremely short lives always bursting suddenly and unexpectedly with a loud bang. Children over about 7 years old will not take analogies so literally, and the kind of military terms often used can be very successful to explain, for example, the body's defences.

Lastly, it is clear from the above description of stages that health professionals are not faced with an enormous variety of explanations of medical events, but with a systematic developmental progression. Yet as Bibace and Walsh (1980) point out, children's books on illness and hospitalization appear to be based on an adult's construction of how children think, rather than on empirical data revealing how children do think. With regard to health professionals, Perrin and Perrin (1983) asked paediatricians, nurses and child development students to estimate the age at which children made typical responses to five questions regarding illness mechanisms. Clinicians usually overestimated the age of younger children and underestimated the age of older children; they correctly estimated children's ages less than 40 per cent of the time. The findings of this study supported the conclusion that:

Physicians and nurses make little use of the notion of developmental stages, and approach all children more or less as if they were in middle childhood, or in the Piagetian stage of concrete operations.

A similar study of nurses' knowledge of children's conceptualisation of illness also found that nurses' knowledge was limited in some areas (Rushforth, 1996). One of the reasons for this state of affairs may be that much of the research in this area describes the various stages in a child's understanding of illness, yet gives little practical guidance on the implications for practice. It is possible, however, to state some implications for practice, which can be used when explaining hospital and illness to children.

- There are important differences between the way children understand what they experience and the way adults understand the same experiences. These differences are not haphazard, but can largely be predicted from the child's stage of development. A working knowledge of the various stages of cognitive development (as outlined in this chapter) will help nurses to explain various aspects of illness and hospitalization in a way that will mean something to children.
- Children at the sensori-motor stage (under 2 years) can best be communicated with through their parents.
- Under 7 year olds cannot see the relationship between medical procedures and cure; they are likely to think painful or unpleasant treatment is a punishment for being naughty and will need reassurance that it is not.
- Under 7 year olds find it hard to imagine internal mechanisms in the body and are only interested in what will happen to the body surface, the bit they can see. The important aspects of hospital to children at this stage are observable things, equipment, lights in the operating theatre, food, nurses' uniforms and surface wounds, rather than explanations of what is going on inside the body. Even 9 year olds find it difficult to speculate about what may be going on under the body surface, and it is helpful if explanations can be related to what they can see and touch.
- Over 12 year olds show a growing concern about internal disease processes, and are capable of imagining the sinister implications of pain. They also can foresee being an adult, and the implications of chronic illness (such as juvenile arthritis) can be very upsetting for them. Children at this stage will much appreciate an opportunity and encouragement to discuss such worries.
- The ages given for the various stages are very approximate. It has often been suggested that, when dealing with adults, information gathering should be put before information giving. This is even more important with children. Before embarking on any explanations, it is best to listen first to the child's own explanation. With children, always start from where they are.
- Before talking to children, think carefully about the possible implications of the words used, avoiding potentially frightening words like 'cut', or ambiguous ones like 'organs'. For children over 7 years, it is normally appropriate to use analogies (such as germs as the 'baddies', antibodies as the 'goodies' fighting the battle for health). Younger children tend to take analogies too literally, making them at best confused and at worst very frightened.

Atkinson, R.L., Atkinson, R.C., Smith, E.E., Bem, D.J. and Nolen-Hoeksema S. (1996) *Hilgard's Introduction to Psychology*, 12th edn, Harcourt Brace, Fort Worth.

Beales, G. (1983) The child's view of chronic illness. *Nursing Times*, 79(51), 50–1.

Bennett-Johnson, S. (1988) Psychological Aspects of Childhood Diabetes. *Journal of Child Psychology and Psychiatry*, 29(6), 729–38.

Bibace, R. and Walsh, M.E. (1980) Development of children's concept of illness. *Pediatrics*, 66, 912–17.

Brewster, A.B. (1982) Chronically ill children's concepts of their illness. *Pediatrics*, 69, 355–62.

Bryant, P.E. (1974) *Perception and Understanding in Young Children*, Methuen, London.

Donaldson, M. (1986) *Children's Minds*, Fontana, London.

Goodall, J. (1994) Thinking like a Child about Death and Dying, in *Caring for Dying Children and Their Families*, (ed. L Hill), Chapman and Hall, London.

Greig, A. (1997) Play, Language and Learning, in *Early Childhood Studies: an Holistic Introduction*, (eds J. Taylor and M. Woods), Arnold, London.

Johnson, B. (1990) Children's drawings as a projective technique. *Pediatric Nursing*, 16(1), 11.

Jolly, J. (1981a) *The Other Side of Paediatrics*, Macmillan, London.

Jolly, J. (1981b) Through a child's eyes: the problems of communicating with sick children. *Nursing*, Series 1(23), 1012–14.

Ley, P. (1988) *Communicating with patients*, Croom Helm, London.

Marteau, T.M. (1989) Health beliefs and attributions, in *Health Psychology: Processes and Applications*, (ed. A.K. Broome), Chapman and Hall, London.

Millstein, S.G., Adler, N.E. and Irwin, C.E. (1981) Conceptions of illness in young adolescents. *Pediatrics*, 68(6), 834–9.

Nagy, M. (1952) Children's ideas of the activity of germs. *Health Education Journal*, X, 15–20.

Norbeck, J.S. (1981) Young children's ability to conserve facial identity when facial emotion varies. *Nursing Research*, 30, 329–33.

Perrin, E.C. and Gerrity, P.S. (1981) There's a demon in your belly: children's understanding of illness. *Pediatrics*, 67, 841–9.

Perrin, E.C. and Perrin, J.M. (1983) Clinicians' assessments of children's understanding of illness. *American Journal of Diseases of Children*, 137, 874–8.

Pontious, S.L. (1982) Practical Piaget: helping children understand. *American Journal of Nursing*, 82(1), 114–17.

Rushforth, H. (1996) Nurses Knowledge of How Children View Health and Illness. *Paediatric Nursing* 8(9), 23–6.

Swanwick, M. (1990) Knowledge and control. *Paediatric Nursing*, 2(5), 18–20.

Taylor, J. and Müller, D. (1995) *Nursing Adolescents: Research and Psychological Perspectives*, Blackwell, Oxford.

Turner, J. (1984) *Cognitive Development and Education*, Methuen, London.

Donaldson, M. (1986) *Children's Minds*, Fontana, London.
    Concentrating on a critique of Piaget, Donaldson tells the interesting story of experiments (such as the policeman experiment described here on page 58) which have led us to question some of Piaget's claims, as well as those which

have built on his original view of cognitive development to give us a much clearer idea of how children think.

Oates, J. and Sheldon, S. (eds) (1987) *Cognitive Development in Infancy*, Psychology Press, Hove.

This series of papers provides wide reading around cognitive development, including cross cultural aspects and works on memory and cognition.

Taylor, J. and Müller, D. (1995) *Nursing Adolescents: Research and Psychological Perspectives*, Blackwell, Oxford.

This book includes sections on adolescent cognitive development in relation to health and illness.

CHILDREN AS INDIVIDUALS

5

Chapters 1–4 have emphasized the different ways in which children are comparable to other children and, from this, we have been able to discuss children in a general rather than a specific way. Yet commonsense tells us that children are individuals, and experienced mothers testify to the uniqueness of their infants even from birth. We derive security from feeling that we are different from others and yet remain the same person, even though our appearance may change and our opinions, beliefs and values may alter with time. It is rather strange then that psychologists often seem to describe us in terms of our similarities rather than our differences. We consider in this chapter some aspects of individuality.

INDIVIDUAL DEVELOPMENT

Physical growth charts typically represent weight as a smooth curve of average or normal weights, but this disguises the sudden spurts and intervening plateaux of individual children. Figure 5.1 shows the weights of sisters born at the same time of year, two years apart, and starting off with almost identical weights. It is possible to see that their growth patterns are very individual. One might think from much of the material presented in the previous chapters that all infants and children develop psychologically at the same rate and in the same way. Many infant and childhood abilities are described in relation to age but, while a child of 4 years of age may be able to do many more things than a child of 2 years, two children of the same age may be unable to do the same things. It is

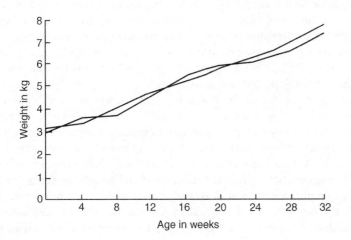

Figure 5.1

Graph to show growth by weight of sisters born two years apart (from data collected by one of the authors from children in Norfolk),

not age, as such, which defines the various limits of ability. Chapter 4 shows how Piaget used the more general term 'stages' to demonstrate that, although there is a typical sequence to childhood development (i.e. the development of thinking and reasoning), it is the sequence rather than the specific age which is important.

Another way in which children vary is in their response to experiences. For example, in Chapter 2 the problem of developmental delay in children in institutions was mentioned (Dunn, 1980). What is interesting is that the delay did not occur in all children; although they shared the same impoverished environment, only some appeared to suffer from adverse effects.

An important issue in research into individual differences in children concerns the social context of development. It is difficult to say with certainty which characteristics in an individual are inborn and which have developed as a result of interaction with other people and the world around (Rutter, 1985). Some children can be seen to behave very differently in the presence of a grandparent or the father, compared with the mother with whom much of the research into child psychology has been conducted. It is also worth bearing in mind that, when adults are interacting with children, it is not just the children who are changing and developing. Adults react to life changes (e.g. marriage, occupational stress, menopause or retirement) and though events may have little if anything to do with the relationship with the child, they may nevertheless affect it. In terms of researching and trying to measure individual differences, the intrinsic characteristics of a particular individual can be extraordinarily difficult to identify amongst a myriad of interpersonal experiences.

Another factor related to the social context, which may affect the study of individuality, is the experience of the situation in which behaviours are seen. It was found in one early study described in Tyler (1978) 'that children can be readily induced to think in a style they do not spontaneously employ' (p. 157). The study was concerned with disadvantaged black children, and showed that by encouraging active participation in a sorting task (e.g. making up groups of everyday objects such as a cup, ball, top, pencil, bottle opener) the children became generally more flexible in their ability to solve problems. If they were only allowed passive participation, such as explaining the links between the items which had been sorted into groups by someone else, then the flexibility in thinking did not occur.

Not surprisingly then, research has been conducted with very young children and infants in an attempt to minimize the effect of experience but the original hope of psychologists to be able to measure pure native characteristics which have not been contaminated by stimulation, experience or training has not found fruition. Indeed Simonoff *et al.* (1994) suggest that trying to understand behaviour in terms of pure heredity or pure environment is a false distinction. The important point is how the two interact. Scarr and McCartney (in Berger, 1985) actually suggest that experience itself is directed by genotype which raises some interesting questions. Berger (p. 5) writes that Scarr and McCartney's theory:

> *attempts to account for the processes whereby individual differences in responsiveness to environment influence the nature of the experience which a child both undergoes and creates.*

STUDYING INDIVIDUALITY

Much of the research on early development has concentrated on describing what babies can do. Chapter 2 summarizes much of this work. However, although babies' abilities are impressive, the effect of this approach is to generalize development rather than trace the particular developmental patterns of individuals. In the study of individuality, the reverse is true. Here, we are especially concerned with the ways in which individuals develop. For example, in general, wariness of strangers is noted in infants about the age of 6 months. This is a useful rule of thumb, but it is important for nurses to know that it is not true of all babies. Dunn (1979) describes some research which identified signs of wariness in some babies at 4 months of age. What is interesting about this though is that such babies had also shown a particular pattern or style of reacting to other experiences at even younger ages. They had been more upset and startled by being bathed, or seeing a suddenly looming object, than other babies. This longitudinal study of infants suggests that from a very early age they already have an individual 'style' of behaviour. Compared with others they are wary of certain experiences and, though they do the same things as other babies, they are distinguishable from them by the way they behave.

In studying individual differences, various attempts have been made to distinguish between what individuals do in terms of their general developmental ability, and how they do it. Words such as 'style' or 'patterns' of behaviour are used to help us appreciate the differences between individuals. During the 1960s, Thomas, Chess and Birch became renowned for their research into individual styles of behaviour. Their particular contribution to this field was the longitudinal study of many individuals from infancy through to early adulthood. Longitudinal research is difficult for several reasons and psychologists often prefer to undertake cross-sectional studies. For example, if a researcher decided to measure children's honesty from the ages of 5 to 15 years, he could do so by once a year giving them a questionnaire suitable for their level of understanding. This research would take more than 10 years to set up, conduct and analyse. Meanwhile the children's families might move away, or the researcher might encounter all sorts of other difficulties in locating them. To make life easier, the research could be done in a year by selecting groups of children in each age bracket who are matched for details such as sex, social background, culture and so on. In a cross-sectional study like this the researcher would have one result for each child, but a number for each age group. It would therefore be possible to see how children's honesty in general changed with age, but not how individuals changed. To find this out, the much more time-consuming longitudinal study would need to be conducted.

Interestingly, when research into children's honesty was carried out with a sample of several thousand children (Hampson, 1982) it was found that individual children were not consistently honest, but were influenced by situations, so they would be honest sometimes but not always, and different children were honest over different situations. This individual variation is also subject to a general developmental consideration: children do not develop mature moral thinking to enable them to be consistently honest across a variety of situations until at least early adolescence (Hampson, 1982). This suggests that the study of individual differences should be carried out, bearing in mind the generalized findings of developmental psychology. But if the long term study of individuality is so difficult why do some psychologists think it is important?

One reason may be the deeply rooted belief that early experience affects later behaviour and personality development (see Chapter 1). It is widely believed that deviance and illness could be prevented or minimized if we knew what to look for in the early years to predict problems later. Thus, by comparing observations of behaviour in early life with later outcomes, particular behavioural styles which seem to be maladaptive could be identified and the knowledge used to try and prevent similar problems in others. At first this idea sounds very promising, but the future is not totally predictable and infancy, childhood and adolescence are not necessarily just preparatory stages for later development. Wolkind and Rutter (1985) and Rutter (1985) made the important point that just because psychologists have shown that a particular behaviour occurs, say between a mother and child, it does not automatically mean that this behaviour is actually important in the long run. Baltes *et al.* (1980) suggest that earlier stages of development are preparatory to a degree only. To understand development properly it is, they say, legitimate to examine the stages as described by Piaget (Chapter 4), for example, as well as the whole lifespan. Full understanding of the implications of either is dependent on a detailed knowledge of both.

PREDICTING DIFFICULTIES

Individual differences are found in various human attributes: physique, activity levels, skills and interests (e.g. musical, sporting, artistic), academic ability, sociability, emotional behaviour, the way we sleep, express tension, and even in the way we think. Individuality, though, does not only apply to 'normal' or 'healthy' people. Although it is common to categorize disabled people according to their disability, Birchenall (1995) reminds us of the importance of highlighting the abilities and potential of individuals. Regardless of ill health or disability we all have the right to have our unique individuality recognized.

The work of Thomas *et al.* (1963, 1968) concentrated on investigating individual differences in temperament and personality. By analysing questionnaires completed by parents of infants and young children, the researchers were able to identify certain behaviours, which appeared at an extremely early age, relating for example to activity level, regularity of body functions such as eating and bowel movements, and quality of mood. These were found to cluster together in different ways in different children. For instance, a child who was described as having a positive mood, regular bodily functions and being adaptable, was regarded as an 'easy' child. On the other hand, 'difficult' children were intense in their reactions, irregular in body functions, and slow to adapt, with a negative mood. Thomas *et al.* wanted to try and see if behaviour patterns in infancy and childhood were useful as predictors of later behavioural disturbance, and if behaviour patterns were stable over time. It was found that only the very extreme individuals presented behaviour which could in any sense predict later problems. While some children who became psychiatric referrals displayed particular 'difficult' behaviour patterns, many more children later presented for psychiatric help than had displayed the behaviours which were thought to be useful as predictors. What was also interesting was that behaviours in the first year of life were no different for those needing psychiatric intervention later on than for the rest of the group. However, during the second year, temperamental characteristics did correlate with the children needing help. Further follow-up of this longitudinal study (Thomas and Chess, 1982) also found significant correlations between temperament at 3 and 5 years of age and early adult temperament.

These results suggest two things: firstly, that early behaviour is not a particularly good predictor of later outcome, and secondly that temperament is not always stable over time, especially the first two years. Interestingly, this is a period when much research into individual differences is carried out partly because, as mentioned earlier, it is assumed that environmental and interpersonal influences will have less of a confounding effect on the results. Underlying biological considerations may be important, and it has been thought that studying young children may reveal the differences attributable not to environment or experience, but to genetic endowment and biological factors.

BIOLOGICAL CONSIDERATIONS

Many books and articles written about individual differences discuss the role played by genetics in making children different. However, it is surprisingly difficult to be sure whether behaviour is determined genetically. For example Dunn (1980) describes cross-cultural studies comparing American and Mexican-Indian babies. The American babies cried more intensely and slept more deeply, while the Indian babies stayed longer in a quiet alert state. These findings could be due to genetic, environmental, or caregiving differences. Similar differences were experienced by Schmitz *et al.* (1995) in their attempts to estimate the relative importance of genetic and environmental influences on problem behaviour in children. What becomes increasingly apparent is that genetics and environment are closely linked in development in what Plomin (1995) describes as a 'duet relationship' rather than with one directing 'the performance' of the other. For example, children with a genetic disposition to be tall cannot realize their full growth potential unless their nutrition (an environmental factor) is sufficient.

A typical approach in studying temperamental differences is to study twins who are genetically identical, having formed from the same cell (monozygotic twins). The idea is that because they are genetically identical, any differences between them must be due to environmental influences. Research by Torgerson (1982) tends to support the idea that genetic factors influence some aspects of the development of temperament, but not that temperament is necessarily inherited.

Another example of research which relates to the biological context is described in Hampson (1982). In a large longitudinal study concerned with the development of social behaviours such as dependence, aggression and achievement, it was discovered that during the period from infancy through early adulthood, boys and girls differed in respect of aggression, dependency and passivity. While aggressive behaviour in boys of 6–10 years of age correlated with their aggressiveness as adults, this was not so with girls. On the other hand, girls had stable patterns of dependency and passivity over a similar time period, while boys did not. The children's development as individuals was subject to this more general sex difference, but it was not possible to say whether changes they experienced in relation to aggression, dependency and passivity were due to biological maturation, socialization, or a combination of both.

PERSONALITY AND INTELLIGENCE

Two topics which have also yielded results applicable to the study of individual differences concern personality and intellect. 'Personality' is a word which probably implies to many people the distinguishing features of a person; those which make a person different from anyone else. This has been discussed in Wattley and Müller (1984), with examples of questionnaires and rating scales which have been used to try and measure personality. All the measures were designed for adults, but it is also possible to design them at a suitable level for children. Eysenck (1965) modified an adult version which measured traits such as extraversion and neuroticism to form a Junior Personality Inventory. Other examples of personality measures for school children of different ages are Cattell's *High School Questionnaire, Children's Personality Questionnaire* and *Early School Personality Questionnaire*.

The work by Eysenck has shown that extraversion is stable enough to be reliably predicted for adolescents from their childhood scores. Leiderman (1989) found that nearly all personality factors measurable in adults can be found in children. In reporting the research in this area, Hampson (1982) points out that the evidence suggests continuity of personality factors across age-groups, but there may be variations in the actual scores. Thus, extraversion may score high at one age and low at another. The trait remains, but its significance may vary from time to time in the same individual.

The study of intellect in psychology has a very long history. Tyler (1978) has pointed out that its attraction originally lay partly in the fact that children at the turn of the century were gradually becoming subject to the common experience of education, which emphasized reading and counting. Thus researchers could, at least crudely, find large groups of children who to some extent could be said to be experiencing similar types of stimulation and learning experience. Although intelligence is difficult to define, various measures designed by different psychologists seem to produce similar results, and intelligence test results invariably seem to correlate with school success. However, it is easy to think of intelligence as relating only to academic or school ability, since high scorers do well in these fields. Others who may not score highly in school-type tasks may be excellent swimmers, mechanics, musicians, cooks or artists, and it is important to recall that people differ as to which skills they learn readily and which they find difficult.

Among earlier work on children's individual differences in intelligence were studies of gifted children. In summarising this work, Tyler (1978) reports that such people, studied longitudinally through childhood into adulthood, were always to be found achieving more than the less gifted, and very few became failures. Thus their high intelligence as tested in school did seem to be predictive of high achievement in society as adults. In contrast, other people who had seemed more delayed with regard to school achievement also averaged lower on indices of success and achievement in later life. However, they were still mostly able to be self-supporting, marry and have children who were doing satisfactory school work themselves. As Tyler points out, intelligence tests test 'schoolability' not the ability to survive or adapt to the practical circumstances of life. In contrast, a more recent review by Freeman (1995) of the current findings of several international longitudinal studies found that the gifted children were no more likely to be high achieving adults than others who were randomly selected from similar social and economic backgrounds.

When more ordinary children are tested longitudinally regarding intelligence, some interesting trends occur. At one stage a child may appear to be developmentally delayed, but then suddenly show rapid improvement before levelling off. Similarly another child may repeatedly score above, then below, average from one year to the next. Another pattern which Tyler (1978) describes is the child who scores extremely highly in nursery school and then drops slightly but steadily downwards. This indicates the importance of longitudinal studies, otherwise we might assume that ability at one age is stable for life and fail to appreciate a child's changing needs and developmental status. The research in general suggests that bright children generally remain bright, and dull children generally remain dull. Large changes in either direction are unusual, but smaller changes in either direction are common. Again we return to the genetic–environmental debate in this discussion. Freeman (1995) suggests that 70% of intellect is genetically determined, leaving 30% which is open to environmental influences. Small but significant changes in direction are attributable to the 'individual way of organising and using knowledge in an adaptive goal-directed way, which is heavily dependent on the social and educational environment' (p. 536).

THE CONTEXT OF INDIVIDUALITY

Although research into intelligence or personality as an indicator of individual differences is interesting, it is also narrow and tends to miss the point now emerging in research into this field: that it is not the individual components of a person (e.g. personality or intelligence) which determine a person's individuality, so much as what Berger (1985) calls 'activity'. In the course of a person's life, choices have to be made about which stimuli to respond to, which alternative to act on, or which codes to live by. The range of choices at any moment is phenomenal, and it increases with age, mobility, experience, resources and factors relating to personality, intelligence and so on. What we are measuring when looking only at intelligence is one component which will exert an effect in combination with many others to determine a person's individual uniqueness. To be able to nurse children as individuals, it is not enough to know that in general children of a certain age like to play in same-sex groups, or can conserve measures of volume and see who has the most orange juice to drink. We, as nurses, need to be able to discover whether a child in our care does show these preferences and skills, and to see them as only part of a whole comprising numerous experiences unique to each child.

If we take this kind of approach, it becomes less important to know details such as whether the same personality trait is being manifested consistently over time in one child. Instead it is more important at any given moment to consider the interaction between the child's range of individual characteristics, past experiences, the opportunities provided by the environment, and the interactions between the child and various others, especially the usual caregivers. It appears that children who have a combination of those factors which suit them are likely to do well. Children who have an unsuitable combination do not (see Rutter (1985) for further discussion).

To avoid maladjustment, it is not sufficient to identify a single causal link relating to, for example, personality, caregiving styles, relationships or intellect. The potential to develop optimally requires that children's individuality be recognized through and within the constellation of experiences, interactions and personal characteristics unique to each child. There is no single formula which, if applied to all children, would ensure their optimum development.

It is important to realize the contribution that children themselves make to the experiences which may shape their development. In particular, children often affect how other people respond to them (Freeman, 1995) and this in turn may affect the range of a child's life experience. While attentive mothers seem to have responsive babies (Wolkind and Rutter, 1985), alert babies receive more attention from their mothers. Similarly, Dunn (1980) describes a newborn nursery where active babies received more attention from the nurses. Clearly these babies may enhance their opportunities of experiences through interaction.

We saw in Chapters 3 and 4 how important experience is for early development. On the other hand, however, children with certain traits may experience an escalation of difficulties because their behaviour makes their mothers tense. Dunn and Kendrick (1982) found this to be so in children who exhibited traits such as an above average 'negative mood' and 'intensity of emotional expression' prior to the birth of a sibling. When the new stressor appeared, these children became more withdrawn, or had sleep problems, or became very clinging. This led to more confrontation with the mother, though it was not shown that these problems were permanent.

As was mentioned, it is important to remember that children, their parents and their nurses are all developing independently of each other in relation to their own lives and life events and in response to each other through interaction. This means that development in and between individuals is a dynamic process rather than a static and unchanging situation. When we consider the children in our care, we should realize that we too play a part in the process of the development of their individuality.

INDIVIDUAL DIFFERENCES IN PERSPECTIVE

In Chapter 1 we pointed out how assumptions rather than scientifically tested knowledge can affect or govern practice. This can be true of our views about newborns being treated in sex appropriate ways (e.g. blue and pink blankets), or of our views on parental presence in the anaesthetic room. Although we intuitively feel that people do differ from each other, and although we may prize and even guard our own individuality, it is often quicker, apparently more efficient, less demanding and possibly considered more just to treat everyone the same. On the other hand, it sounds very humane to talk of treating people as individuals. We made a case in Chapter 1 for discovering the research bases of professional practice. In the case of children as individuals, this means examining the research evidence to see if they differ in measurable ways. If we find that they do, we may be presented with a clash of needs: the hospital may appear to demand efficiency by treating everyone in the same sort of manner. The nurse in turn may feel that this is preventing focus on the needs of the individual. What then are the conclusions to be drawn from this chapter as they apply to nursing?

Evidence is very clear that children are different from each other.

They show this in all sorts of ways, such as activity level, emotionality and sociability. However, especially in infancy and early childhood, it is difficult to show that particular characteristics remain the same in a particular child. Rather, children's optimum psychological development seems to be dependent upon a combination of factors: the child's own characteristics, the environment and their interactions with others. A good combination can enhance the likelihood of children realizing their developmental potential, but a poor combination can lead to maladaptive behaviour. This is difficult to predict because there are so many variables involved. It is interesting that this theme concerning combinations of factors has appeared again. It has already been mentioned in earlier chapters in relation to the experience of separation and hospitalization, that children who came from backgrounds with enduring problems, or who were faced with a number of problems at one time, were far more likely to be disturbed by a strange event than others for whom a single stressful event occurred.

Two main points arise from the study of children as individuals. One is that there is no psychological support for the idea that children should be treated in the same way. Not only do they need different approaches, but also they themselves unconsciously elicit different approaches from their caregivers. It would be reasonable to ask caregivers to develop awareness of the ways in which they themselves react, noting both to whom they react, and why; and whether there are individual children who tend to be overlooked. The second point follows on from the first. It is that sensitivity to the constellation of factors affecting each individual child is important if health care professionals are to be able to understand the children in their care as individuals and meet their individual needs. Dunn (1980, p. 108) puts this succinctly:

> ...it would be deeply misleading to imply that by identifying a child's temperamental characteristics we could predict developmental outcome with any certainty. Understanding the course of development means taking into account the complexity of mutual influences over time, the social and cultural environment of the family, the stresses to which it is exposed and so on.

These findings may cause nurses to reconsider the values which govern practice in their wards and departments, and to assess whether their aims are to focus on the child as an individual. In nursing we talk a great deal about individualized care but what we talk about is not always translated into practice. It would be interesting to consider what assumptions and values govern current practice and to determine what is our shared understanding of individualized care. As Price (1996) writes:

> Belief in children as individuals with specific needs, combined with the adoption of a philosophy or model of care, is not sufficient to ensure individualized care. Such beliefs have to be combined with a system of organizing nursing work that enhances their effectiveness.

◀ In practice

- There is no single correct way to treat all children. Nurses and midwives need to develop sensitivity to the nature of each child's individual characteristics and relate them to the child's own world.
- Children behave differently in the presence of different people, which may include nurses. This could be useful in situations where a child responds well to a particular person who could then be involved in helping a child cope where unpleasant treatments have to be given to the child. Similarly, it might be wise to avoid putting particular nurses with children who apparently do not respond well to them.
- Some children put themselves in an advantageous position developmentally by attracting attention through being alert or active. Others may not, and caregivers should try to be aware of which individuals are more easily overlooked, especially if they are unable to benefit from the environment as a result.
- Nurses, parents and others are themselves developing as individuals. It is important to remember this when working alongside each other. Different situations will affect different individuals in different ways and nurses need to be sensitive to this in others and aware of it in themselves.

REFERENCES

Baltes, P.B., Reese, H.W. and Lipsitt, L.P. (1980) Life span developmental psychology. *Annual Review of Psychology*, **31**, 65–110.

Berger, M. (1985) Temperament and individual differences, in *Child and Adolescent Psychiatry*, 2nd edn, (eds M. Rutter and L. Hersov), Blackwell Scientific Publications, Oxford.

Birchenall, M. (1995) Disability: An Issue for the Growing Child, in *Childhood to Adolescence: Caring for Health*, (ed. A. Fatchett), Baillière Tindall, London.

Dunn, J. (1979) The first year of life: continuities in individual differences, in *The First Year of Life. Psychological and Medical Implications of Early Experience*, (eds D. Shaffer and J. Dunn), John Wiley, Chichester.

Dunn, J. (1980) Individual differences in temperament, in *Scientific Foundations of Developmental Psychiatry*, (ed. M. Rutter), Heinemann, London.

Dunn, J. and Kendrick, C. (1982) Temperamental differences, family relationships and young children's response to change within the family, in *Temperamental Differences in Infants and Young Children*, (CIBA Foundation Symposium), Pitman, London.

Eysenck, S.B.G. (1965) A new scale for personality measurement in children. *British Journal of Educational Psychology*, **35**, 362–7.

Freeman, J. (1995) Recent Studies of Giftedness in Children. *Journal of Child Psychology and Psychiatry*, **36**(4), 531–47.

Hampson, S.E. (1982) *The Construction of Personality. An Introduction*, Routledge & Kegan Paul, London.

Leiderman, P.H. (1989) Relationship disturbances and development through the life cycle, in *Relationship Disturbances in Early Childhood*, (eds A.J. Sameroff and R.N. Emde), Basic Books, New York.

Plomin, R. (1995) Genetics and Children's Experiences in the Family. *Journal of Child Psychology and Psychiatry*, 36(1), 33–68.

Price, S. (1996) Concepts of Individualised Care, in *Children's Nursing*, (eds L. McQuaid, S. Huband and E. Parker), Churchill Livingstone, New York.

Rutter, M. (1985) Psychopathology and development: links between childhood and adult life, in *Child and Adolescent Psychiatry*, 2nd edn, (eds M. Rutter and L. Hersov), Blackwell Scientific Publications, Oxford.

Schmitz, S., Fulker, D.W. and Mrazek, D.A. (1995) Problem Behavior in Early and Middle Childhood: an Initial Behavior Genetic Analysis. *Journal of Child Psychology and Psychiatry*, 36(8), 1443–58.

Simonoff, E., McGuffin, P. and Gottesman, I.I. (1994) Genetic Influence on Normal and Abnormal Development, in *Child and Adolescent Psychiatry: Modern Approaches*, 3rd edn, (eds M. Rutter, E. Taylor and L. Hersov), Blackwell, Oxford.

Thomas, A. and Chess, S. (1982) Temperament and follow-up to adulthood, in *Temperamental Differences in Infants and Young Children*, (CIBA Foundation Symposium), Pitman, London.

Thomas, A., Chess, S., Birch, H.G., Hartzig, M.E. and Korn, S. (1963) *Behavioural Individuality in Early Childhood*, New York University Press, New York.

Thomas, A., Chess, S. and Birch, H.G. (1968) *Temperament and Behaviour Disorders in Children*, New York University Press, New York.

Torgerson, A.M. (1982) Influence of genetic factors on temperament development in early childhood, in *Temperamental Differences in Infants and Young Children*, (CIBA Foundation Symposium), Pitman, London.

Tyler, L.E. (1978) *Individuality: Human Possibilities and Personal Choice in the Psychological Development of Men and Women*, Jossey-Bass, San Francisco.

Wattley, L.A. and Müller, D.J. (1984) *Investigating Psychology: A Practical Approach for Nursing*, Harper & Row, London.

Wolkind, S. and Rutter, M. (1985) Separation, loss and family relationships, in *Child and Adolescent Psychiatry*, 2nd edn, (eds M. Rutter and L. Hersov), Blackwell Scientific Publications, Oxford.

FURTHER READING

Paton, D. and Brown, R. (1991) *Lifespan Health Psychology: Nursing Problems and Interventions*, Harper Collins, London.

Rutter, M., Taylor, E. and Hersov, L. (eds) (1994) *Child and Adolescent Psychiatry: Modern Approaches*, 3rd edn, Blackwell, Oxford.

For those who may wish to read in greater depth about individual differences, this large collection of papers makes interesting reading.

PART TWO

CHILDREN, HOSPITALIZATION AND HOME CARE

CHILDREN AND HOSPITAL – A BRIEF OVERVIEW 6

In Part One we looked at child development and, in particular, those aspects of development which are of most importance to nurses as they carry out their duties with children. In this part, discussion is concentrated on the child and adolescent in hospital, and on alternatives to hospital care. It will be seen that many of the negative effects found by researchers, which are discussed in Chapter 7, can be avoided by careful preparation, and by sensitive management within hospital. These two themes are the focus of Chapters 8 and 9. Chapter 10 looks at the very special needs of the adolescent in hospital and the theme for Chapter 11 is community child care, which is a rapidly developing area.

In the first chapter of this part, however, we focus on the early work of nurses, doctors, psychologists and indeed parents who provided much of the impetus for the changes which have occurred in the care of sick children over the last 50 years. Some of this work involved the scientific study of children, whilst other work arose from intuition, anecdote and the observation of individual children in different settings. The accumulation of these various sources of data brought about a revolution in the care of children and their parents in hospital. It must be recognised, however, that the revolution was not an easy one for those pioneering for change. They fought an establishment which was steeped in traditions, routines, and regimens, not only regarding the care of children in hospitals but also regarding the place of children in society, their rights and the rights of their parents.

A CLIMATE FOR CHANGE

None of the advances which were made in the care of children in hospital could have happened if the ideas proposed had not occurred in a receptive climate. The changes which did occur must therefore be placed within the context of public opinion at the time, and public opinion was running very high towards the end of the Second World War and in the post-war years. In 1944 Lady Allen of Hurtwood raised the plight of deprived children in a letter to *The Times* and in 1945 the death of a child, Dennis O'Neill, further raised questions in the minds of the public. Dennis had been boarded out (fostered) by a local authority and subsequently died of neglect and ill treatment. In 1946 *The Curtis Report* was published, having been set up to inquire into existing methods of providing for children who were, for whatever reason, deprived of a normal home life with their parents or relatives and 'to consider what further measures should be taken to ensure that these children were raised in conditions best calculated to compensate them for the lack of parental care'.

During the same period a number of professionals were also beginning to ask questions about the effects of deprivation and separation upon children. Dorothy Burlingham and Anna Freud, directors of the Hampstead Nurseries, which provided care for children who could not be cared for in their own homes during the war years, observed that even in these nurseries, where the levels of care were far superior to the care in large institutions, the children were delayed in aspects of development including speech, toilet training and control of aggression (Burlingham and Freud, 1942, 1944). Similar observations were made in a number of papers published during the war debating the effects of evacuating children against the effects of air raids, including such titles as *The Bed-Wetting Problem* (Miller, 1940) and *The Effects of Evacuation and Air Raids on City Children* (Burbury, 1941). The consensus of opinion at the time was that, on the whole, children who remained in the air raids with their parents fared better (psychologically) than those who were evacuated without their parents. This point was emphasised in the *New Statesman* in 1941 by an entry in a poetry competition which won second prize (Cited in Bowley, 1958, p. 194).

> *I wanna go home, this place is plumb dead,*
> *I'd rather be blasted to bits,*
> *And enjoy mi own dirt, wi'aht stockings and shirt,*
> *It's home, and who cares for the blitz?*

So far, however, the debate about separation from parents had focussed on residential nurseries and foster homes and the care of children in hospitals had escaped attention. Not for long though. James Robertson, who had worked with the staff at the Hampstead Nurseries had, along with John Bowlby, been awarded a grant in 1948 to undertake inquiry into the effects on personality development of separation from the mother during the child's early years. Robertson observed a number of children who had been admitted to hospital. His observations included both the period of hospitalization as well as the period after the children had been returned home, and he recorded his observations in a remarkably moving film – *A Two Year Old Goes to Hospital* (Robertson, 1952). The film is still widely available and should, in our opinion, be essential viewing for any student. Film was of course a popular medium during and after the war, and Robertson's work documented the emotional stages through which children pass when separated from their parents in hospital. These stages included protest, despair and detachment, as well as the difficulties that children and their parents experienced after they returned home.

Bowlby was equally if not more influential, and had been asked by the World Health Organization in 1950 to advise on the mental health of homeless children. His findings were published the following year. Bowlby described 'the prevalence of deplorable patterns of institutional upbringing and the crass indifference of certain hospitals to childish sensitivities ...' (Bowlby, 1951). In 1953 he published a further influential text in which he described complete maternal deprivation where a child is removed from his mother and there is no *one* person who provides care in a personal way and with whom the child feels secure. He cited much evidence to support the effects of deprivation upon these children who, he felt, would almost always be physically, intellectually and socially retarded. He suggested that children under the age of seven years would be affected the greatest. The effects of the deprivation would, he believed, persist into adulthood.

The work of Bowlby and Robertson in the early 1950s (Bowlby, 1969; Robertson and Robertson, 1989) provided the impetus for others to study the effects of separation on the child. These publications included: *Deprived Children* (Lewis, 1954), *The Normal Child* (Valentine, 1956), *The Magic Years* (Fraiberg, 1959) and *The Psychological Effects of Hospitalization in Infancy* (Schaffer and Callendar, 1959). Professionals and the public alike became concerned over the short term effects of separation as well as the long term, permanent effects of being separated from parents. Fraiberg (1959, p. 293) wrote, for example:

> *Children who spent their infancy and formative years under these conditions revealed the effects of an impoverishment of the personality, as if a nutritional deficiency had affected the early structures and devitalized parts of the personality . . .*

It was further thought that these children would, in later years, find they were unable to have adult relationships with others and would be unable to 'love deeply, to feel deeply . . .'. Others added to the debate. For example, Schaffer and Callendar (1959) studied infants and their reactions to separation and concluded that, although babies under 7 months of age were not unduly upset by hospital and responded to the nurses when their mothers left them, they were quieter when they returned home and mothers found it difficult to re-establish previous contact with their babies. Later research was to refine and elaborate upon this early work, and indeed focus upon the resilience of children as opposed to their emotional weaknesses. However, at the time in post war Britain it was very influential and very disturbing.

THE EFFECTS ON CHILDREN'S SERVICES

To say that the work of the psychologists and others was welcomed by those who were charged with looking after children in hospital would, however, be a gross exaggeration! Many hospitals, including children's wards (although many children were cared for on adult wards), were run along almost military lines. Spence, in a famous lecture which was published in the *British Medical Journal* in 1947 gives a vivid description of what it was like:

> *A white-coated young man arrives and descends upon the silent occupant of a bed who, knowing that her penicillin hour is at hand,*

breaks her silence in a four-hourly scream. There are other distractions at other times – the daily or twice-weekly promenade of an older man in black with a retinue of followers; the occasional quick incursion of a young man more sprucely clad, who pronounces his decision with a 'put him on the list for next Tuesday'; the solemn visit of the matron, who passes from bed to bed with the same question on her lips at every bed; the arrival of an injured child at night; the piece of chocolate after dinner; the excitement of strange instruments which the doctors and nurses use but do not explain. Night comes on but there is no bedtime story, no last moment of intimacy, no friendly cuddle before sleep. The nurse is too busy for that ...

Visiting times were, in most cases, subject to strict rules which could not be broken and often completely ruled out children having any regular contact with working fathers whilst in hospital. Visiting was generally prohibited on 'operating day', meaning that children might have no contact with a parent for up to 48 hours at a very traumatic time in their lives. For children unlucky enough to be in hospital when an outbreak of a communicable disease, such as measles, occurred they could be prevented from seeing their parents for several weeks. Pearce (1949) describes how the ward would be closed to visitors and new patients and no patient would be discharged or moved from the ward for any purpose. Operating would be suspended. This type of quarantine would persist until no new cases had occurred for two weeks. However, if a new case occurred the quarantine arrangements would begin again. Similarly, the importance of a strict regimen was the order of the day in terms of bringing up children at home. Truby King in the fourteenth edition of his book *Mothercraft* (1943) insisted that routine was all important in bringing up a baby, saying that 'his education begins from the very first week, good habits being established which remain all his life' (p. 4). Evelyn Pearce in *A General Textbook of Nursing* (1949, p. 274) also highlights this:

Between the age of 18 months and 2 years the child ought to be taught to speak correctly, to walk, to control and regulate micturition, to have regular habits of bowel evacuation, to wash his hands before eating and to clean his teeth.

He requires regular meals and regular sleep. A child of this age usually wakens about 6 a.m.; he should immediately empty his bladder, and may have a drink of water or milk and water; he must stop in bed without disturbing other people until 7.15, but he may have a toy to play with or a book to turn over the pages. At 7.15 he will be washed and dressed ready for breakfast at 8 o'clock. After breakfast he should immediately have an action of the bowels before play or other interest can be entertained. He may play and be amused until 10.30 when he should be put to rest in his perambulator in the open air. He will sleep for an hour or more, but

he may not get up until 12 noon, when he should empty his bladder,
be washed and prepared for dinner at 12.30.

However, change did happen, in spite of resistance. First, the famous Dr Truby King had died and, in spite of others taking his work forward, his place as the guru of parentcraft was taken over by Benjamin Spock who published a number of widely sold books on baby and child care and the problems of parenthood. His work was easy to read and permitted parents to be more flexible and responsive, and allowed them to give way to feelings of frustration, and indeed to acknowledge they had feelings too. His work includes reference to his own children and those of his friends and was a huge contrast to the dictatorial writings of Truby King. For example, in one chapter entitled 'The Whiner' in *Dr Spock Talks with Mothers* (1961) Spock wrote 'I remember, many years ago, when I went to an all-day picnic with another family, being driven nearly mad by the continual whining of their five-year-old-son and – even more – by the patient way in which the mother let it go on' (p. 147). Spock also mentioned, in the same book, how children may see illness as a punishment and blame mothers for failing to provide protection against painful procedures. He emphasized how important it was to spend time with ill children in hospital.

Another change, first introduced by Spence in Newcastle upon Tyne, was the admission to hospital of mothers with their sick infants. This initiative was followed by Sister Ivy Morris and Dr Dermod MacCarthy in Amersham in the 1950s (Burton, 1997). The Amersham scheme attracted media attention (and some ridicule!), but was pivotal in encouraging other units to follow suit. In 1958 Robertson made a second film *Going to Hospital with Mother* (Robertson, 1958) which featured the Amersham unit and was as powerful in contrast as the film *A Two Year Old Goes to Hospital* published six years earlier.

The third event, instrumental in bringing about change, was the publication of *The Platt Report* in 1959 which made far reaching recommendations about, among other things, visiting and added official recognition to the views of those psychologists, nurses and doctors who had been campaigning for so long.

Finally, the formation in 1961 of *Mother Care for Children in Hospital* – a group of mothers from London who came together after seeing Robertson's films, and two years later the formation of the NAWCH added the voices of parents to the campaign for change.

THE LARGE INSTITUTIONS

Although progress was slowly being made to help children admitted to a general hospital and their parents, and further research was being carried out, for one group of children life did not look so hopeful. These were the many children admitted each year, and residing in, the large institutions built for the 'mentally retarded'. Furneaux (1973) and Edgerton (1979) both describe the situation in these institutions at the time when children's units were becoming much more liberal. Furneaux (1973, p. 172) suggested:

> *to sit in the ward and savour the squalor and horrible stench of the communal potting session is a test of endurance … what must these children … be enduring who have known differently but who, because nothing else is available, have to live as members of such a community and take part in such activities?*

In 1962, however, the British Psychological Society undertook a large survey which covered some 30 per cent of the total admissions to the large institutions in England and Wales. It also highlighted the fact that, for many of the children admitted, the institutions were not suitable, but they were there because there was no alternative (British Psychological Society, 1966).

In 1964, Jack Tizard tried an experiment in which he removed 16 severely mentally retarded children from a large institution and placed them in smaller family type units. He studied their development and found that, when matched with controls who had remained in the large institution, the children in the smaller unit had improved in their verbal and social development as compared with the control group. It was finally being appreciated that children with learning disabilities were also suffering from the deprivation described in other children ten years earlier which finally led to changes in this sector of the health services too.

To conclude this chapter, which we hope provides some background to the rest of this part, we would add a note of caution. It is 50 years since it was first proposed that separating children from their parents caused short and possibly long term distress for children and we have focussed upon some of the very early work which took place in the 1940s, 1950s and early 1960s. Further work was undertaken throughout the 1960s and 1970s and yet, as you will read in subsequent chapters, it was not until the mid 1980s that resistance to change finally seemed to disappear and policies on unrestricted visiting became universal – some 40 years after Dorothy Burlingham and Anna Freud made their first observations.

REFERENCES

Bowlby, J. (1951) *Maternal Care and Mental Health*, WHO, Geneva.

Bowlby, J. (1953) *Child Care and the Growth of Love*, Penguin, Harmondsworth.

Bowlby, J. (1969) *Attachment and Loss* Penguin, Harmondsworth.

Bowley, A. (1958) *The Natural Development of the Child*, 4th edition, E. and S. Livingstone, Edinburgh.

British Psychological Society (1966) *Children in Hospitals for the Subnormal*, Report of the British Psychological Society.

Burbury, W.M. (1941) Effects of Evacuation and Air Raids on City Children. *British Medical Journal*, 660.

Burlingham, D. and Freud, A. (1942) *Young Children in War-time*, Allen and Unwin, London.

Burlingham, D. and Freud, A. (1944) *Infants without Families*, Allen and Unwin, London.

Burton, V.M. (1997) The origins of open visiting and resident mothers at Amersham Hospital. *Journal of Child Health Care*, 1(2), 78–80.

Curtis, M. (1946) *Report of the Care of Children Committee* (Curtis Report), HMSO, London.

Edgerton, R. (1979) *Mental Retardation*, Fontana/Open Books, London.

Fraiberg, S.H. (1959) *The Magic Years: Understanding the Problems of Early Childhood*, Methuen, London.

Furneaux, B. (1973) *The Special Child*, 2nd edn, Penguin, Harmondsworth.

King, M.T. (1943) *Mothercraft*, 14th edn, Whitcombe and Tombs Limited, London.

Lewis, H. (1954) *Deprived Children*, Oxford University Press, London.

Miller, E. (1940) The Bed-Wetting Problem. *Mental Health*, 1(1).

Pearce, E. (1949) *A General Textbook of Nursing*, 10th edn, Faber and Faber, London.

Platt, H. (1959) *The Welfare of Children in Hospital: Report of the Committee on Child Health Services*, HMSO, London.

Robertson, J. (1952) *A Two Year Old Goes to Hospital* (Film).

Robertson, J. (1958) *Going to Hospital with Mother* (Film).

Robertson, J. and Robertson, J. (1989) *Separation and the Very Young*, Free Association Books, London.

Schaffer, H.R. and Callendar, W.M. (1959) Psychological Effects of Hospitalization in Infancy. *Journal of Paediatrics*, **24**, 528.

Spence, J.C. (1947) The Care of Children in Hospital. *British Medical Journal*, I, 125.

Spock, B. (1961) *Dr Spock Talks with Mothers: Growth and Guidance*, The Bodley Head, London.

Tizard, J. (1964) *Community Services for the Mentally Handicapped*, Oxford University Press, London.

Valentine, C.W. (1956) *The Normal Child and some of his Abnormalities* Penguin, Harmondsworth.

7 THE EFFECTS OF HOSPITALIZATION ON CHILDREN

Why is that one child will sail through a hospital stay with only the occasional apprehensive moment while another, admitted for exactly the same reason, will be desperately unhappy throughout? Is it something to do with each child's past experiences? is it something one child's parents have done that the other child's parents have omitted to do? What other factors might affect the way a child responds to hospitalization? And, the most important question of all, can nurses do anything to minimize unhappiness on their wards? Before we can attempt to answer these questions, we need to look at the nature of adverse reactions to hospital, both during the hospital stay and after discharge from hospital. We can then look at those factors in the parents and children which affect how they react to hospital, and lastly at those factors which are a part of the hospital experience itself that have been shown to affect responses to a hospital stay.

ADVERSE REACTIONS TO HOSPITAL

Visintainer and Wolfer (1975) classified the features of hospital which could worry a child into the five categories below, each of which has implications for management.

1. Physical harm or bodily injury in the form of discomfort, pain, mutilation, or death.
2. Separation from parents and the absence of trusted adults, especially for pre-school children.
3. The strange, the unknown and possibility of surprise.
4. Uncertainty about limits and expected 'acceptable' behaviour.
5. Relative loss of control, autonomy and competence.

It is worth noting that these are the kinds of worries that would also affect adults in a hospital situation. Visintainer and Wolfer (1975) were comparing the effects of different forms of preparation on the reactions of children during hospitalization. Their classic study, which is still referred to frequently in the literature, is described in some detail here since it not only demonstrates some of the problems involved in assessing children's reactions to hospital, but also indicates the types of responses that are indicative of stress.

Two measures of children's emotional states were taken, and their level of cooperation rated on five occasions during hospitalization – the admission examination, blood test, pre-operative medication, transport to the operating theatre, and while waiting in the foyer of the operating theatre. The observers also noted any resistance to the anaesthetist. The first measure was the 'manifest upset scale', a five-point scale intended to reflect the child's emotional state in terms of verbal and nonverbal expressions of fear, anxiety, or anger. The scale took into account the amount of energy the children put into their response (e.g. a soft cry indicated less upset than screaming) and the activity required to control the upset (e.g. upset that could be controlled by verbal comfort or verbal restraining was less than that requiring physical comfort or physical restraint). A 'frozen' or panic response was considered to show extreme upset. A rating of one point indicated little or no fear or anxiety, and a rating of five points indicated extreme emotional upset.

The second measure, that of cooperation, was also rated on a five-point scale and was intended to indicate the degree to which the child cooperated with a procedure. A rating of one point indicated complete cooperation, including active participation in, and assistance with, the procedure, and a rating of five points indicated extreme resistance, strong avoidance and the necessity to restrain the child. In addition, Visintainer and Wolfer (1975) quote interesting evidence showing that the more emotionally upset a patient is, the more medication is required, the more difficult it is for the patient to take drinks, and the longer it is before the patient passes urine. On the basis of this evidence, they decided to use recovery room medication requirement, ease of fluid intake and time to first passing urine as further measures of children's reactions.

Analysis of these measures revealed that all the children showed varying degrees of upset, with the younger children (under 6 years) having significantly higher upset ratings, showing significantly less cooperation than the older ones, and finding it more difficult to drink. It is possible that the greater amount of distress in the younger children was in part affected by the methods used to assess that distress. Apart from the 'frozen' response (which was given a high distress rating), *manifest* upset is the criterion used and it is likely that older children would be less likely to show their distress in such obvious ways. Whatever the precise interpretations of the results however, one finding remains clear: the experience of hospital is, to varying degrees, a stressful one for children.

Short term effects

Looking at the short term effects once the child has been discharged from hospital, Cross (1990) followed the progress of 50 children aged between two and seven years at weekly intervals following discharge. Her results showed that 54 per cent of children experienced difficulties when they returned home. Common behavioural problems were increased nervousness about separation, demanding behaviour, sleeping difficulties and difficulties with mother–child and sibling relationships. It would be interesting to investigate whether there is a correlation between those children whose parents were resident throughout their stay and separation anxiety.

On the other hand, McClowry and McLeod (1990) in a study of 50 school-age children (aged 8–12 years) found there were no significant behavioural differences following discharge. Their findings lend support to other researchers (including Visintainer and Wolfer, 1975) who have found that older children cope with the experiences of hospital without demonstrating negative behavioural changes. McClowry and McLeod, in attempting to interpret their findings, discuss several possibilities. Primarily, children of this age group could be resilient to the stresses of hospitalization. Secondly, children of this age are able to disguise their behaviour so that it does not reflect their feelings. Mothers would be unable, therefore, to perceive any changes. Thirdly, that the measuring tool was not reliable and finally, that the perspective was too narrow. They suggest a broader approach which encompasses attributes such as the severity of the illness, the personality of the child and the existing family situation. Support for this approach was provided by correlating variables relating to these areas. These variables are discussed later in the chapter.

Long term effects

What about long term effects? Robertson and Robertson (1989) in an account of their influential work in this field describe in vivid detail the long term effects of hospitalization on children. Their work began in the 1940s when children with tuberculosis often spent several years in long stay institutions seeing their parents for limited periods of time each week. The Robertsons followed many of these children into adulthood and noted the difficulties they had in adapting to social norms.

Parmelee (1989, p. 159) also discusses the effects of acute physical problems that lead to hospitalization:

> *The potential for long term interference with the development of normal relationship concepts as a result of these major acute events is evident.*

Parmelee places the blame for post-hospital problems firmly at the door of the parents, saying that they may overemphasize the physiological needs of the child even after he or she has recovered, which causes conflict within the child who is ready and able to resume usual activities. On the other hand, Fletcher (1981, p. 192) in his review of such research, concludes:

> *It seems safe to say that children who have been reported to exhibit psychological upset post hospitalization usually return to their pre-hospital levels of behaviour within the first 6 months after discharge.*

A study by Peterson and Shigetomi (1982), which followed up 40 children one year after tonsillectomy operations, suggests that past concerns about long term emotional trauma may be unwarranted. Their interviews documented a tendency for children to recall more positive than negative aspects of hospitalization, and the authors suggest that this indicates the possibility of psychologically beneficial results of a child's hospitalization experiences. Harris (1979) also found evidence of beneficial reactions to hospitalization, mainly in terms of greater confidence. Much of the research evidence for within hospital and post-hospital upset is contradictory and confusing, partly because there are so many factors which will contribute to the reaction of any individual child. Bolig (1984, pp. 325–6) concludes:

> *With the information provided by more than 40 years of cumulative data, social scientists and practitioners clearly recognize that hospitalization is an inherently stressful experience for children and their families. Most children as well as many adults, evidence symptoms of distress while hospitalized ... Children may be more resilient than earlier believed, and brief, isolated hospitalizations may not be necessarily 'traumatic'. Nevertheless, hospitalization must be considered a 'crisis', as both opportunity and danger exist for coping, adaptation and continued learning.*

The remainder of this chapter discusses specific factors which appear to be important in terms of what makes children react in the way they do.

FACTORS IN PARENTS AND CHILDREN AFFECTING REACTION TO HOSPITAL

Much of the research looking into the effects of hospitalization has attempted to identify why different children react to their experiences in different ways. For example, Visintainer and Wolfer (1975) attempted to relate hospital upset to one or more specific characteristics of the 'consumers' of hospital. They were unable to produce clear evidence in support of this view. Cross (1990) also looked at factors which could correlate with children who were upset. Her only significant finding was that, after the age of five, children settled at home much more easily than younger children. Jolly (1989), in her discussion of construct theory and adaptation to hospitalization, emphasizes the importance of the child's personality. She found that children who are 'well adjusted' are likely to experience fewer problems than children who are not. Again, she does not produce clear evidence to support this correlation.

Hall (1987) in his review of social and psychological care before and during hospitalization warns of the dangers of concentrating on specific factors within the child. For example, he states that if hospitals concentrate on reducing disturbances in the younger age groups it could be to the detriment of older children who may be equally disturbed but do not demonstrate their distress so overtly. Hall emphasizes (on p. 723) the need to take a much broader perspective, while still recognizing the potential influence of certain factors:

> *A more generalised model of hospitalisation distress can be built around concepts of vulnerability and coping behaviours, stress and*

mastery, and dis-equilibrium and discontinuity, in which age and developmental maturity are important variables, along with family lifestyle and hospital environment and experience. The concepts are interrelated.

It would appear, therefore, to be much more productive to take a flexible approach in looking at the characteristics of parents and children which will affect their reaction to hospital; what appears to be important are not the *stable* characteristics of the people concerned, but rather a mixture of past and present experiences, feelings and expectations.

Previous separation experiences

Whilst great strides have been made to reduce separation when children are in hospital, such as open visiting and free accommodation for parents, it is naïve and inaccurate to assume that all parents have the resources to be able to stay with a sick child throughout his or her stay either because of work commitments, or because they have other children to care for, or because they are in hospital under police protection. It is these children who spend some or all of their time in hospital unaccompanied who are the focus of the following discussion.

One issue discussed frequently in the literature is the effects of previous separation experiences on the child. This issue is complex and there appear to be many conflicting viewpoints (Deater-Deckard *et al.*, 1996). It is, however, important to discuss these here because of the implications for nurses working with children.

The early work of Bowlby and the Robertsons (cited in Robertson and Robertson, 1989) discussed the detrimental effects of separation on children. However, in their latest research the Robertsons concluded that not all children would suffer and that 'variables do play a large part in determining the young child's response to separation'. They do not discuss evidence which suggests that children in hospital will react to their experience differently if they have had previous separation experiences but do identify that the child's relationship with the parents will affect behaviour. Deater-Deckard *et al.* (1996) in a study of children separated from parents through day care and their subsequent behaviour also found that a number of variables will influence the child's experience of separation, in particular the home environment, maternal stress and parenting.

Roggmann *et al.* (1994) reviewed the growing body of research relating to children who have been separated repeatedly from their parents and their subsequent attachments. Their meta-analysis of research showed few effects. The view that children who are frequently separated from their mothers during their first year may be more likely to develop insecure attachments is inconclusive although it is possible that a correlation could exist between frequency of separation and reaction to separation. There is obviously a need for further research into this area before accurate conclusions can be drawn.

What if the previous separation actually involved a hospitalization?

Again there appears to be conflicting evidence about whether this has an effect on behaviour. There is growing evidence to suggest that one operation does not prepare children in a positive way for all others. Children who have had surgery before tend to be *more* anxious than those experiencing surgery for the first time (Crocker, 1980).

Cross (1990) found that there was no significant difference in behaviour between children who had been in hospital fewer than five times and those in for the first time. However, children who had six or more previous admissions were significantly more unsettled. Asthmatic children appeared to have more difficulty coping than other groups of children. Interestingly, Cross found that none of the children who were admitted for surgery experienced behavioural problems following discharge. It is difficult to interpret this finding as no correlations between diagnosis and previous admissions, or diagnosis and mode of admission (emergency, 24 hour notice and waiting list) were made.

McClowry and McLeod (1990), in their study of school-aged children, found no relationship between previous hospital admissions and behavioural disturbances.

Other stressful experiences prior to hospitalization

Crocker (1980) notes that events such as the birth of a sibling, the death of a pet, a move to a new house, a new or first school, or a family fight, coupled with hospitalization can create more stress than the child can handle. Berden *et al*. (1990) also discuss the effects of major changes within the lives of children and the subsequent stress on the child. Most children are able to cope with infrequent stress but major or long term stress can have negative effects. If children are suffering from stress prior to their admission to hospital it could affect their ability to cope with the further stress of hospitalization. Hall (1987) suggests that children can be helped to cope with stress by giving them practical and emotional support. The occurrence of a recent upset in a child's life may therefore suggest to ward sisters or charge nurses that the timing of elective admissions should be delayed where possible and, in emergency cases, sensitivity may be needed in order to help children cope with their stress.

Symptoms

Another aspect of the previous experiences of hospital consumers is the symptoms the child has exhibited prior to hospitalization, which naturally affect both the child and parents. It is certainly worth considering the possibility that younger children may be extremely confused by their medical treatment if they have not experienced any unpleasant symptoms. It is hard for a child to understand how pain and separation are supposed to make him or her feel better, but if there had not even been any obvious illness the negative aspects of hospital would presumably be doubly difficult to take.

Cross (1990) in fact found that children admitted from the waiting list showed fewer behavioural problems than children who were admitted as emergencies. However, many other variables were not accounted for which could have influenced these findings, such as preparation for admission, the presence of parents and whether or not the child had symptoms.

A study by Harris (1979) included both an asymptomatic group and a group with fairly disabling symptoms, but the presence of disabling symptoms made no difference to the children's desire for a 'cure'. It appears that children have other reasons for wanting to obtain a correction of their condition, and that suffering unpleasant effects plays only a small part in the way they view the necessary medical treatment. All these children, however, were old enough to understand that there may be other unpleasant effects of illness besides pain or discomfort. It would surely be worth explaining to younger children with asymptomatic conditions exactly why they need treatment.

Parents' feelings about hospital

The role of parents in their children's reaction to, and recovery from, illness and hospitalization is frequently emphasized in the literature, and here we discuss how parents' attitudes towards hospital can influence both their own and their children's reactions. In an early study, Robinson (in Stacey, 1970) asked mothers whether or not they had been hospitalized under 5 years of age, and also what they remembered about it. His hypothesis was that a mother who remembers being upset by hospitalization would be more likely to want to accompany her child into hospital, to prevent upset in her child. This hypothesis was supported; the mothers who had been upset as child patients were more likely to say that they would live in. However, interestingly, when it came to the *actual* visiting (as opposed to the *intention* to visit), those mothers who visited most were those with the least fear of hospitals. Those with a high personal fear were more ready than those with less fear to prepare a child before, and outside, the hospital situation. A further effect of mothers' fear of hospital was a reluctance to come into contact with hospital staff, and an unwillingness to admit that they were dissatisfied with any aspect of the hospital situation.

Robinson also looked at the effect of a mother's fears on her perception of her child's fear. His data supported the theory that the arousal of fear in one person results in a tendency for that person to also perceive other people as fearful and anxious. The 'fearful' mothers in Robinson's study were more likely to be concerned about their own child being frightened than mothers who held no fears about hospital. This is an important finding, since the 'fearful' mothers' attitudes could lead to a self-fulfilling prophecy; children could see that their mothers expect them to become frightened, and therefore they too became frightened. They might also think 'Mum thinks I'm going to be scared, so there must be something here to be scared of'. Other studies have also looked at parental attitude and temperament and the physiological status of the child. For example, Garrison *et al.* (1990) showed that temperament of the mother was related to metabolic control in a study of children with insulin dependent diabetes and a study by Carswell *et al.* (1990) discusses the relationship between parental stress and control of asthma in children. If nurses contribute to parental stress, therefore, they may be unwittingly causing further distress to the children in their care.

Previous mother–child relationship

Not all children fret when they are separated from their mothers, and it would be tempting to suggest that this is because they do not have a particularly good relationship with their mothers anyway so they do not miss them when separated. Early researchers did in fact suggest this. It appears that the issue is not clearcut however, since Emde (1989) found that short term distress is *less* if the child has a good relationship with the mother and the mother is emotionally sensitive and responsive to cues from the child. The only reasonable conclusion we can come to is that the quality of the mother–child relationship *is* an important factor in how a child reacts to separation, but whether it improves or worsens the reaction depends on what the separation *means* to the child. As we have seen in Chapter 3, the reaction varies as the child develops.

FACTORS AT THE TIME OF HOSPITALIZATION

In this final section we look at those characteristics of the hospital experience itself, which have been shown to affect the risk of upset in children and parents; these are: duration of hospitalization; presence of parents in hospital; staff–parent relationships.

Duration of hospitalization

Cross (1990) in her study of 50 children following discharge found no significant relationship between length of stay and behavioural difficulties. These findings are different from those of Douglas (1975) who, on the basis of his analysis of data on 3000 children, claimed that children who have to go into hospital for more than a week before the age of 5 years are more likely to develop problems as teenagers, manifested chiefly as behaviour disturbance and poor reading. Single hospital admissions of a week or less were not associated with an increased risk of disorder in adolescence. Although the findings indicated an association between prolonged or repeated hospital admissions in early childhood and an increased risk of behaviour disturbance in adolescence, care needs to be taken in interpreting such results in too simple a way (longer hospitalization leads to greater risk of post-hospital disturbances). Children experiencing longer hospitalizations are likely to have more serious illnesses with more pronounced physiological effects. Frequent lengthy hospitalizations such as are common with chronic illness (see Chapter 12) change a child's life in a number of ways. Therefore we cannot conclude that, on its own, the length of hospitalization has any direct effect on reaction.

Presence of parents in hospital

We now reach an area which has been talked and written about more than any other aspect of children in hospital in recent years. This is the effect on the child of the parents' presence in hospital.

The Platt report (1959) recommended that parents should have unrestricted access to their children in hospital. Action for Sick Children (previously The National Association for the Welfare of Children in Hospital) has consistently campaigned for this goal and monitored the effects of such campaigning. In 1982, a NAWCH survey which looked at access on children's wards throughout England was undertaken by Thornes (1982). The survey found that progress was slowly being made and 49 per cent of wards studied allowed unrestricted access for parents. The survey also looked at where children were being nursed and found that despite the recommendations of the Platt report (1959), 28 per cent of children were still being nursed on adult wards. Whilst it might have been anticipated that the parents denied open access to children were those whose children were being nursed on adult wards, the survey showed that 48 per cent of children's wards still did not have open access. The children who fared worse were children on ear, nose and throat wards with 24 per cent being denied visits on the day of operation and with many spending up to 36 hours away from their parents.

A follow up study by NAWCH (1986) showed a great improvement, although a detailed look at changes in the interim year showed a few instances where small children's units had closed and children transferred to adult wards. NAWCH warned that 'we all need to be very vigilant'. The second survey was, however, on the whole very encouraging with 85 per cent of parents having open access and another 4 per cent open access except on operating day. In 1993 the Audit Commission showed further improvement but highlighted the particular needs of adolescents (see also Chapter 10). The success of the NAWCH campaign has resulted in the organization raising awareness about other issues (Rice 1988).

> ...the work has become more subtle. No longer is it mostly removing physical barriers but more to do with changing staff attitudes if parents are not made welcome.

Staff–parent relationships

It is to this issue that we now turn our attention. While the NAWCH (1986) survey showed that most parents are allowed open access, the same report estimated that although 67 per cent of parents were welcomed on wards, 24 per cent were merely 'accepted' and 9 per cent were 'tolerated'. These estimates of attitude were subjective and research which correlates quality of care with the degree to which parents are welcomed has not, to our knowledge, been carried out.

Why is it then that parents are not welcomed onto wards? One possibility could be the system of care delivery and the influence of the ward sister. A comparison of two ward sisters (Brown 1989) noted that the sister who ran a system of task allocation on her ward was less welcoming than the sister who practised patient allocation. The 'task' sister, when asked to describe her ward at its most ideal, was reported to say:

> When it's empty. When everything is running smoothly, and this depends on the age group of the children and whether the parents are sensible or not.

Brown clarified the sister's definition of 'sensible' parents. They were parents who 'respected the nurses' and made 'nice comments' about them. Taylor (1996) also discusses that nurses do have 'popular' and 'unpopular' families (a point highlighted by Stockwell in 1972 in relation to adult patients). Reading these studies, a picture emerges of problems of empowerment and of families receiving differential levels of care apparently at the discretion of the nursing staff. Neatness and tidiness were also a worrying aspect of Brown's study. This is totally opposed to what Fradd (1986) describes as a successful and welcoming child care unit where 'permission to make a "mess" (is) essential' or what Ainsworth (1989) described in her account of a unit which goes one step further and also welcomes pets.

Without doubt, the advantages of having open access for parents and welcoming their presence on the ward outweigh the disadvantages. It must be said, however, that nurses involved in the care of children in hospital have had to adapt their role (Taylor, 1996; Bishop, 1988). Bishop (1988, p. 61) writes:

> It would be silly to deny there are disadvantages to having parents participate in care. But most appear to be related to nurses' attitudes. Some are concerned about the loss of structured routines and fear that the numbers of parents will interfere with the running of the wards. Fear, also, of loss of traditional nursing practice, loss of formality, and loss of control, play a part in the reluctance to changes in practice.

The advantages of welcoming parents to our hospitals are best illustrated by looking at the studies of the care-by-parent units, where parents are taught to provide 24 hour care but are able to have access to nursing care if required. Cleary et al. (1986), in their study, which compared children in the care-by-parent unit with children with a resident parent and children without a resident parent, showed that the children in the care-by-parents and resident parent groups spent significantly less time alone and cried less and had less contact with non-family members, while parents had more discussion time with doctors. On the other hand the children in the group without resident parents were cared for by 'an ever changing series of nurses', spent more time asleep, more time alone and more time crying.

Care-by-parents (either in a special unit or in a children's ward) is a far more common occurrence than previously was the case. It is however vital that children's units plan for such participation to occur rather than adopting a 'take it or leave it' attitude. The parents, the child and the health care professionals need to be fully aware of their respective duties, obligations and rights (Palmer, 1993). Building a relationship of trust is clearly crucial if parents are to have a 'caring partnership' with professionals. Parents must be given information about what is happening to the child (Long, 1997; Kristjansdottir, 1991). If parents are to participate in care they need to have clearly defined roles so that they know what is expected of them. Family centred care can only be realized if parents are fully aware of what they are supposed to be doing. Nurses who are interacting with parents who are caring for their own children in hospital also need to be aware of the many ways in which parents may behave when they are anxious and how they can develop their own interpersonal skills to provide optimum support (Farrell, 1995).

Before concluding this section on the presence of parents in hospital it is important to mention one further point. The needs of parents in hospital are important and nursing staff should ensure that they get adequate rest, regular meals and that their other basic needs are met (Palmer, 1993; Long, 1997). The NAWCH (1986) survey looked at accommodation and facilities for parents and concluded that facilities needed to be improved, as did the Audit Commission (1993) who found, for example, that one-third of wards had no facilities for parents to wash or shower.

The need for clarity was highlighted in a study by Webb *et al.* (1985) which showed a significant discrepancy in procedures that parents perceived they would be capable of performing and those which nurses thought they would be able to perform. This study highlights the need for careful planning and evaluation of care. Parents should negotiate in this process so that everyone concerned in the 'partnership' (for example, child, parents, nurse, physiotherapist) has an awareness of the others' roles. As with any change process it is important that the needs of those involved are not overlooked. Nurses need to be prepared for their changing role (Palmer, 1993), especially those nurses who find it difficult to accept the changes within the environment and their role with parents. It will also be necessary for administrative changes to take place. A recognized place is required, a parents' 'territory' near to the ward, both for practical and symbolic reasons, establishing their right to be there. A DHSS (1984) circular states:

A sitting room should be available for parents and relatives who will need somewhere to relax and have beverages; this guidance assumes that parents and relatives will take main meals in the staff dining room. The room should be pleasantly furnished with tables and comfortable chairs and should be planned within easy reach of the bedrooms.

Just as importantly, nurses too require a 'retreat' so that they are not permanently on view or within earshot of parents.

From the studies we have looked at, it seems that any changes necessary are fully justified by the advantages of parents having unrestricted access to their child. These include the reduction of the trauma of separation and hospitalization, the child being able to go home sooner if the parents have instructions on how to provide care while in hospital, reduction of postoperative complications and, lastly, the contact with other parents which can provide much needed support. There are two other aspects of the hospital experience which have been shown to affect reaction to hospitalization. The first is preparation of children and parents for the events of a hospital stay, which is such a large topic that the whole of Chapter 8 is devoted to this. The second aspect is the effect of hospital procedures and the hospital environment on a child's reaction. Treatment procedures and the environment in which they take place are an integral part of the care of the child in hospital, and are further discussed in Chapter 9.

◄ In practice

- Children coming into hospital are likely to be worried about being physically hurt, being separated from known and trusted adults, facing the unknown, and feeling uncertain about how they should behave. Older children are likely to fear loss of control and independence in much the same way that adults do. They need to be assured that such fears are perfectly normal, and verbal children will benefit from the opportunity and encouragement to talk about their particular worries so that misconceptions can be corrected.

- Children, like adults, do not always show their emotions. They may seem quiet and accepting but, deep down, they may be very frightened. It is wise not to assume that a child is fine just because there is no obvious sign of distress. The encouragement to talk, and perhaps a reassuring cuddle, may be required even when not requested verbally.

- Even when there is little clear evidence of harmful effects of hospitalization, a child's happiness is still a very valid aim. There is ample evidence that the happy child recovers physically in a shorter time and it is therefore well worth trying to make life in hospital as friendly as possible. Chapter 9 outlines a number of ways that this may be achieved.

- Distressing events in a child's life preceding a hospital stay can make the experience of hospital 'the last straw'. If a child has had previous unhappy separation experiences, or important life events, hospital can be too much to cope with. It is worth talking to the child and family to discover if anything outside the hospital stay has proved upsetting to them.

- It is also likely that young children who have experienced no unpleasant symptoms will find treatment particularly difficult to comprehend. These children would especially benefit from careful, sensitive, age appropriate explanations (see Chapter 4) of treatment procedures, to avoid unhappiness within hospital and resentful behaviour difficulties afterwards.

- The presence of parents has been shown to be beneficial to children, both physiologically and psychologically. If parents are nervous or uneasy, their children may sense this and become frightened themselves. Parents need a defined role in the hospital and this may involve nurses showing parents how to care for their children in a way that is medically acceptable while involving a family-centred approach to care. Nurses can, in turn, learn a great deal by watching how parents treat their children.

- Staff and parents need to be able to get along well together and for this to happen both parents and nurses need their own 'territory', a place to which they can retreat and relax.

REFERENCES

Ainsworth, H. (1989) And the guinea-pig came too. *Nursing Times*, 85(39), 54–6.

Audit Commission (1993) *Children First*, Audit Commission, London.

Berden, G.F.M.G., Althaus, M. and Verhulst, F.C. (1990) Major life events and changes in the behavioural functioning of children. *Journal of Child Psychology and Psychiatry*, 31(6), 949–59.

Bishop, J. (1988) Sharing the caring. *Nursing Times* 84(30), 60–61.

Bolig, R. (1984) Play in hospital settings, in *Child's Play: Developmental and Applied*, (eds T.D. Yawkey and A.D. Pellegrini), Laurence Erlbaum, Hillside, NJ.

Brown, R. (1989) *Individualised Patient Care*, Scutari Press, Middlesex.

Carswell, F., Heck, G., Robinson, E., Hallows, D., Peters, T. and Stanton, T. (1990) Family stress and childhood asthma. *Nursing Practice*, 3(3), 10–15.

Cleary, J., Gray, O.P., Hall, D.J., Rowlandson, P.H., Sainsbury, C.P.Q. and Davies, M.M. (1986) Parental involvement in the lives of children in hospital. *Archives of Disease in Childhood*, 61, 779–87.

Crocker, E. (1980) Reactions of children to health care encounters, in *The Hospital Care of Children: A Review of Contemporary Issues*, (eds G.C. Robinson and H.F. Clark), University Press, New York.

Cross, C. (1990) Home from hospital. *Nursery World*, 90(3228), 22–3.

Deater-Deckard, K., Pinkerton, R. and Scarr, S. (1996) Child Care Quality and Children's Behavioral Adjustment: a Four-year Longitudinal Study. *Journal of Child Psychology and Psychiatry*, 37(8), 937–48.

Department of Health and Social Security (1984) *Health Building Note 23, Hospital Accommodation for Children*, HMSO, London.

Douglas, J.W.B. (1975) Early hospital admissions and later disturbances of behaviour and learning. *Developmental Medicine and Child Neurology*, 17, 456–80.

Emde, R.N. (1989) The infant's relationship experience: developmental and affective aspects, in *Relationship Disturbances in Early Childhood*, (eds A.J. Sameroff and R.N. Emde), Basic Books, New York.

Farrell, M. (1995) The Effect of a Child's Hospitalisation on the Parental Role. *Professional Nurse*, **10**(9), 561–3.

Fletcher, B. (1981) Psychological upset in post-hospitalized children: a review of the literature. *Maternal Child Nursing Journal*, **10**, 185–95.

Fradd, E. (1986) It's child's play. *Nursing Times*, **82**(41), 40–42.

Garrison, W.T., Biggs, D. and Williams, K. (1990) Temperament characteristics and clinical outcomes in young children with diabetes mellitus. *Journal of Child Psychology and Psychiatry*, **31**(71), 1079–88.

Hall, D. (1987) Social and psychological care before and during hospitalisation. *Social Science Medicine*, **25**(6), 721–32.

Harris, P.J. (1979) *Children, their Parents and Hospital*, Unpublished PhD thesis, University of Nottingham.

Jolly, J. (1989) The child's admission to hospital. *Nursing*, Series 3(34), 40–42.

Kristjansdottir, G. (1991) Needs of Parents of Hospitalized Children. *Issues in Comprehensive Pediatric Nursing*, **14**(1), 49–64.

Long, S. (1997) Being Together as a family. *Paediatric Nursing*, **9**(6), 25–8.

McClowry, S.G. and McLeod, S.M. (1990) The psychological responses of schoolage children to hospitalization. *Children's Health Care*, **19**(3), 155–60.

National Association for the Welfare of Children in Hospital (1986) *NAWCH Jubilee Review*. *NAWCH Update*, Autumn, 1986.

Palmer, S. (1993) Care of Sick Children by Parents: a Meaningful Role. *Journal of Advanced Nursing*, **18**, 185–91.

Parmelee, A.H. (1989) The child's physical health and the development of relationships, in *Relationship Disturbances in Early Childhood*, (eds A.J. Sameroff and R.N. Emde), Basic Books, New York.

Peterson, L. and Shigetomi, C. (1982) One-year follow-up of elective surgery child patients receiving preoperative preparation. *Journal of Pediatric Psychology*, **7**, 43–8.

Platt, H. (1959) *The Welfare of Children in Hospital. Report of the Committee on Child Health Services*, HMSO, London.

Rice, T. (1988) Caring for children. *Nursing Standard*, **2**(48), 44.

Robertson, J. and Robertson, J. (1989) *Separation and the Very Young*, Free Association Books, London.

Roggmann, J.A., Langlois, J.H., Hubbs-Tait, L. and Rieser-Danner, L.A. (1994) Infant Day Care, Attachment and the 'File Drawer Problem'. *Child Development*, **65**, 1429–43.

Stacey, M. (1970) *Hospitals, Children and their Families*, Routledge and Kegan Paul, London.

Stockwell, F. (1972) The Unpopular Patient, RCN, London.

Taylor, B. (1996) Parents as partners in Care. *Paediatric Nursing*, **8**(4), 24–7.

Thornes, R. (1982) *Parental access and family facilities in children's wards in England*, NAWCH, London.

Visintainer, M.A. and Wolfer, J.A. (1975) Psychological preparation for surgical patients: the effect on children's and parents' stress responses and adjustment. *Pediatrics*, **56**, 187–202.

Webb, N., Hull, D. and Madeley, R. (1985) Care by parents in hospital. *British Medical Journal*, **291**, 176–7.

FURTHER READING   Hill Beuf, A. (1989) *Biting off the Bracelet*, 2nd edn, University of Pennsylvania Press, Philadelphia.
This American book fully explores the social situation of children in hospital. It gives some useful suggestions about improving the psychological care of children.
Taylor, J. and Müller, D. (1995) *Nursing Adolescents: Research and Psychological Perspectives*, Blackwell, Oxford.
Written for nurses, this book is useful further reading for many of the chapters here, but is recommended for this chapter because the Audit Commission has highlighted that whilst many problems relating to the care of children have been, or are being addressed, adolescents are still falling through the net in terms of facilities and care.

PREPARATION FOR HOSPITALIZATION   8

Over the last two decades, great strides forward have been made in recognizing the importance of taking an holistic approach to the care of children. That is not to say that we do not recognize that this sometimes becomes difficult when there are competing pressures on us. In an article on some of the psychological considerations concerning illness and hospitalization, Becker (1980) quotes a senior paediatrician who, having commented on the life threatening nature of many paediatric crises, goes on (p. 11) to say:

> *One simply must attend to these issues as a matter of medical priority, and we often do not have the time and honestly the inclination to intercede on behalf of the best interests of the psychological wellbeing of the child.*

The worrying part about this statement is clearly a lack of inclination on the part of this doctor. Nurses working in children's units also have competing pressures on their time and can easily fall into the routine of dealing only with the physical problems of the child. With shorter and shorter lengths of stay in hospital, the increase in day care and greater pressures on hospitals to increase throughput to reduce waiting lists, it can sometimes feel like we are walking on a treadmill and that there is not enough time to build the scantiest of relationships with one group of children, before they are gone and are replaced with a different group. This is difficult for nurses but does not negate the need to attend to the psychological wellbeing of the children, for however brief the period. We must avoid the misery and sadness of children which has been so vividly described in the past (Hawthorn, 1974; Rodin, 1983; Robertson and Robertson, 1989).

This chapter presents evidence and includes discussion to show how the negative feelings of children can be largely avoided by careful attention to preparation for hospitalization, without encroaching on the staff time required in paediatric crises. In fact, it will be shown that the task of treating children becomes substantially easier if their experiences have led them to trust in staff. The discussion falls naturally into three sections: why prepare, who prepares, and how to prepare.

WHY PREPARE?

Hospitalization has a number of characteristics that can cause children to be very frightened. Several studies have been undertaken which look at the perception children have of hospitals and these give useful information about what aspects of hospitals worry children. Goodman and Adams (1989) asked healthy children to identify words they associate with hospitals. Their response showed that the negative aspects of hospitals were more frequently mentioned with the words smell/disinfectant, fear, anxiety, operation, sad, pain, needles and blood appearing most often. Although their findings did not reach statistical significance, they unfortunately also identified a trend for children who had stayed in hospital to be more negative than those who had not.

Another, small scale, study by Miron (1990) also looked at children's perception of hospital. The children were divided by age into 3–7 year olds and 7–12 year olds. The children in this study identified that nurses were expected to give medicine and be nice. The perception of the younger children of words such as operation, needles and intravenous indicated that the children's knowledge was very limited and in many cases fearsome. In the older age group, the children still perceived operations as being somewhat mysterious although they did at least understand that operations were sometimes necessary to make people better. Many of the older group were aware that people were anaesthetized prior to their operations.

A third study by Price (1988) looked at children's perception of nurses: 203 questionnaires from junior school children were analysed. Results showed that children perceived that nurses would give you stitches and operations and give injections, medicines and pills. Price's study does offer some reassurance to nurses in that, on the whole, the children said very few nasty things about them. The children associated nurses with words such as 'patience', 'kindness' and 'bravery'.

Another potential problem for children in hospital is the number of different people involved in their care. They may, for example, have contact with doctors, physiotherapists, teachers, dieticians, radiographers, domestics, porters, voluntary workers and social workers. They will also meet many new children and their parents. In addition to these people, the children have to contend with the hospital shift system which can bring them into contact with many different nurses. Rodin (1983), in her classic study of children in hospital, reports a description of a child who had 23 complete changes in staff during her stay in an orthopaedic hospital. The so called 'Children's Charter' (Department of Health, 1996) recommends that this should not be allowed to happen, although there are obvious problems in avoiding the multiple contacts suggested by Rodin.

It is clear that children going into hospital meet a large number of different people at a time when, through illness, their capacity for making new relationships is likely to be particularly low. For many children it will be the first time that they have been separated from the cosiness and familiarity of their homes, families and friends, and they may, for whatever reason, also be separated from their parents. In addition, they find themselves in a strange environment where it is hard for them to predict anything, they sleep in different beds, are given different food and often different clothes such as hospital gowns. On top of this, they may be subjected to upsetting, confusing and often painful medical procedures and the very people they have learned to trust and rely on (their parents) may look as worried and confused as they are.

All these factors would be of substantial concern to an adult, but to a child whose understanding is limited by lack of experience and level of cognitive development, hospitalization can be very disturbing. We have looked at children's understanding of illness and hospitalization in Chapter 4, but it is worth mentioning again the work of Miron (1990). She notes that children's immature minds can create disturbing fantasies about what is being done to them, to such an extent that the primary reason for a child's fear is thought to be lack of understanding of medical procedures. The major preoccupations of children coming into hospital are discussed in the third section of this chapter, and in Chapter 9. At this stage, however, it is perhaps sufficient to conclude that hospital has a great deal of potential for inducing fear and unhappiness in its patients. But does preparation help? Eiser (1984), in her review of research on preparation for hospitalization, found it was difficult to isolate any individual aspect that was especially helpful; no single method of preparation had any clear advantage over any other. She writes (p. 184):

> The only consistent finding ... appears to be that any attempts to improve communication with paediatric patients and their parents are better than standard hospital practice.

Similarly, Rodin (1983), in her excellent discussion of preparation for hospital, concludes that children prepared in any way cope better than children who are not prepared.

WHO SHOULD PREPARE?

In the course of her research, Rodin (1983) asked 171 people (parents, paediatricians, paediatric nurses, teachers, playgroup leaders and health visitors) who they thought should tell a child about hospital. Parents were chosen as the most important group of people by 98 per cent of Rodin's sample. Hospital staff can provide accurate information, but parents are needed to interpret that information. Parents know their children better than anyone else, and no amount of knowledge about general child development can completely substitute for the specialized knowledge that is in the possession of a parent, who can relate preparation material in a way familiar to the child. Perhaps a friend has been in hospital recently for similar treatment, or parent and child have watched a television programme about hospitals. Parents are also likely to have more idea of what sort of things worry their child, and this is important information; without it, staff may be telling children what they think they ought to know, rather than discussing what the children have on their minds. On the other hand, Fradd (1996) emphasizes that it is necessary for staff to hear what the child has to say. A parent may interpose answers in order to give a more accurate history, avert criticism, or save the nurses time.

A further advantage of involving parents in preparation is that it reduces discontinuity. In her research, Miron (1990) puts forward the suggestion that social discontinuity between home and hospital may be an important contributing factor in a child's distress in hospital. Having a parent to interpret information and relating it to the child's existing knowledge can reduce the overall strangeness of the situation. However, if parents are to be involved in providing preparatory information for their children, it is important that they should be in possession of the necessary knowledge. Yet those studies that have looked at the information given to parents reveal much dissatisfaction (Ball *et al.*, 1988; Kanneh, 1990; Kristjansdottir, 1991; Eden *et al.*, 1994).

In a study by one of the present authors (Harris, 1981a) the lack of information given to parents caused many to feel frustrated by their consequent inability to answer their children's questions. Nearly all the parents questioned said they had no idea of what their children would face in hospital, and most did not ask. Their main reason for not asking was the consultant's lack of time, implied by the queue of people waiting to see him or her. The problem facing parents in acquiring information was discussed in the Court report (1976), paragraphs 12–25.

A mother who has to spend a prolonged waiting period trying to cope with her ill child and entertain his siblings will most likely be unable to ask sensible questions, or to assimilate information given during the short time she spends with the doctor.

Kiely (1989) found in her study that parents were also reluctant to seek information from the family doctor as this was perceived as bothering them. It appears then that it is unrealistic for nurses to expect all parents willingly to seek information about their child's forthcoming admission. It is important that nurses working in outpatients and in the community are aware of the hesitance of some parents and ensure that information is given to parents without their needing to ask. Nurses in hospital who are involved in the admission of children should recognize that not all parents will be knowledgeable about what is going on. Kiely found that only 42 per cent of parents in her survey had knowledge of admission procedures so it is important that each family is treated individually in order to assess their need for information. The need for parents and children to have information is a key point raised in the 'Children's Charter' (Department of Health, 1996) which tells parents, on page 13:

you and your child have the right to be given an explanation of any treatment proposed including the benefits, risks and alternatives.

Evidence reviewed by Rodin (1983) shows that the anxiety shown by children is clearly and directly related to the anxiety shown by the parent. Glen (1982) points out that when their child is admitted to hospital, parents have many fears, in particular about relinquishing their child's care to strangers and the worry about other children at home. There may be guilt on the part of parents who feel responsible for their child's admission, for example after road traffic accidents, or in cases of child abuse (Chapter 13). Miller (1996) also emphasizes that when a child is admitted as an emergency, the parents often undergo a profound emotional experience and feel very insecure. (Emergency admissions are discussed later in this chapter.) It is also clear that after a child's operation, parents are often worried about their child's chances of survival, even where minor elective surgery is involved. Harris (1981b) asked parents to list the kinds of emotions they felt as their child progressed through the hospital system. Many parents were upset even before admission. The mother of a 5 year old admitted for circumcision said 'I was terribly worried whether he would survive the operation'. Another mother of a 7 year old due to be admitted the next day for orchidopexy said she felt 'very nervous and unsettled'. Nurses who were shown parents' accounts of their emotions were surprised at the sheer intensity of the feelings expressed, particularly as they classed the operations as minor. Parents themselves were also very surprised at their feelings, and it may be useful to forewarn them of the emotions they may experience. To realize that these are neither unusual nor silly (as some parents felt) may make it easier for them to cope with such feelings.

Rodin (1983) points out that in a normal family, children see parents as being in control, providing a framework of security in which they can develop fully and happily. Yet the above research shows that in hospital children may see their parents becoming uncertain and frightened. Preventing this happening is another reason for directing preparation at parents; not only do they need to interpret information, but it is also important that their children should not see them looking uncertain.

Role of playgroups and schools

In preparing a child for hospital, we need to look at the role of playgroups and schools.

In Britain, nearly one million children are admitted to hospital every year. Half of these children are under 5 years old. In addition, over three million children attend hospital accident and emergency departments (NAWCH, 1990; Audit Commission, 1993). Hospitals are therefore all too often a normal part of childhood and, perhaps because of this, the study cited earlier by Rodin (1983) favoured preparation for hospital as a part of general education. Jolly (1981) also feels that hospitals should be included as a subject in the education of all children, not least because under the stress of hospitalization a child's ability to understand may be impaired. She suggests that groups of children should be taken round their local children's ward to see the beds with wheels, bedside lockers, bed tables, curtains round the beds, television, playroom and the nursing staff. She comments that children are often very surprised to know, for example, that a nurse stays awake all night just in case you want her.

Robertson and Robertson (1989), on the other hand, have doubts about this kind of education. They emphasized that young children are very susceptible to fantasy and misunderstanding, and therefore anxiety could be aroused if ideas of separation from home and family, or of pain and mutilation of the body, are introduced unnecessarily. In spite of these reservations, there is some evidence that such preparation can indeed be successful. Rodin (1983) reports on a project where 239 children were visited by three nurses who took medical equipment to their local kindergartens and encouraged the children to play hospital with them. After the play sessions, slides were shown of the hospital and the staff. Subsequently, 78 of the children were admitted to hospital and were found to be less anxious and more cooperative than other paediatric patients. Rodin notes that the programme was later revised so that the school nurse takes over from the visiting nurse, which was seen as making more efficient use of staff time.

How to prepare

What should preparation consist of? A quick answer to this would be whatever a child or parent worries about, but different families will react in different ways to the experiences of illness and hospitalization. According to Crocker (1980), all children need some normality in their routine, opportunities for play and to understand what is happening. These non-medical needs appear to be universal. The age of the child is clearly important. This is fully discussed in Chapter 4, but there is general agreement that the verbal child should be given as honest a picture of forthcoming events as age and development allow. Pre-schoolers understand less in terms of time, and phrases such as 'after your sleep' will mean more to them than tomorrow. Older children will be more concerned with loss of independence and control than with confusing hospital events.

Eiser and Patterson (1984) found that the younger children in their study worried about the physical aspects of hospital (e.g. what a ward looked like, or how a hospital bed differed from their own). Older children talked more in terms of social aspects of the hospital experience such as the role of doctors and nurses in talking to and caring for children, who would visit, and which other children would be there to play with and talk to. All ages recognized that hospitals were associated with pain and discomfort, but older children were more likely than younger ones to mention the social restrictiveness of hospital such as missing school, friends and parents. Eiser and Patterson also emphasize that older children are concerned to be prepared for what is expected of them in hospital.

Besides age, other factors which will influence reaction to any preparatory material include the culture from which the child comes, the reason for hospitalization, the nature of illness and treatment, the amount of contact allowed with parents, level of intellectual development, parents' feelings about the child and about hospitalization, previous surgery, and the child's habitual resources and defences in the face of stress. Perhaps the most important consideration in planning preparation is one that was emphasized some years ago in the Platt report (1959, p. 28):

> *It is never safe to assume that a child will be afraid of an experience*
> *that an adult regards as frightening or conversely that an experience*
> *which has no terrors for an adult will have none for a child.*

Presentation of information

It has already been stated that no one form of preparation appears to have an advantage over any other. In view of all the factors that can affect reaction to preparatory material, it seems that a flexible approach is necessary, and that it varies with the populations, illnesses and medical procedures involved, but always includes a strong component of factual information. However, merely presenting parents and children with information does not necessarily mean that they will absorb it. People can block out unpleasant information, misinterpret it, over- or under-emphasize the importance of particular aspects, and much of whatever information is registered may be forgotten. In their study of parents of children with cancer, Eden *et al.* (1994) found, for example, that nearly ten per cent of the parents could not even remember having an interview with the consultant shortly after diagnosis, and all parents expressed a lack of understanding as to what had taken place. Ley (1988) has done a great deal of work in this area and discusses six ways in which communication of information can be improved:

1. altering the way in which clinicians orally present information to patients;
2. making written materials easier to understand and remember;
3. using illustrations to reinforce written information;
4. making information more readable by the introduction of humour in the form of cartoons;
5. providing patients with a tape-recording of the consultation; and
6. providing access to taped information about the illness and its treatment.

One method Ley suggests, and which is discussed more fully elsewhere (Wattley and Müller, 1984), consists of the nurse presenting information to parents and children in categories which have been announced in advance and thus provide a framework to aid memory. For example, the nurse might say:

> *I am going to tell you – what is wrong with you/your child,*
> *– what tests we are going to carry out*
> *– what I think will happen to you*
> *– what treatment you will need*
> *– what you must do to help yourself.*

The conversation then proceeds with 'First, what is wrong with you ... second, what tests we are going to carry out' and so on. An additional factor to consider in the presentation of information is that a welcoming environment also helps parents and children attend to explanations.

Jolly (1981) emphasizes that learning is incomplete if it relies on the spoken word. It may be enhanced by visual aids but, in her opinion, participation by the child is needed (rather than just listening) if full understanding is to be gained. On this point, Azarnoff and Woody (1981) ask what actually constitutes preparation? Does it include giving written information without seeing that the child and/or the parents read it, or without knowing what their interpretation was? Does it include giving spoken information without observing the response to it? The answer given to these questions is that, ideally, preparation should include methods which actively incorporate the child's and parents' responses and do not simply provide descriptions.

Leaflets and books

Pre-admission leaflets sent by the hospital to elective admissions vary tremendously in quality. Many are not specifically written for paediatric patients and their parents, and very few give information which would help parents prepare their child for hospital. The Consumers' Association report (1980) found that only three-fifths of parents who knew their children were going into hospital received a leaflet beforehand. The most helpful pieces of information were details of visiting times, what to take into hospital and explanations of hospital routines, but in general the leaflets lacked important information. In a later report by the Consumers' Association (1985), they found that hospitals were still not providing relevant information. One child was even advised to bring into hospital a pot to put her dentures in! Very few leaflets give any advice to parents on how they can prepare a child for hospital although Action for Sick Children provide a list of books parents can read with, or to, their children. Their current list is included in the appendix.

The parents in Harris's (1979) study said that they would have liked a comprehensive information leaflet that they could read in their own time, and have an opportunity to ask questions later, for example in the waiting time before admission. A full discussion is given by Harris (1981a) but we list here the information most often requested:

- approximate length of stay;
- day and approximate time of operation;
- detailed clothing and toiletry requirements;
- medical details about the condition (aetiology, treatment, prognosis);
- immediate postoperative effects (sickness? pain?);
- after care;
- hospital routines (what they are, what they are for);
- pleasurable activities available in hospital (e.g. toys, books, video, television);
- a map of the hospital and surrounding area (e.g. places to eat and drink, buy toys, soap, food);

- glossary of medical terms;
- the name of the child's consultant (with pronunciation if necessary); and
- a bibliography of children's books about hospital.

The value of information should not be underestimated. Visintainer and Wolfer (1975) found that for all the children in their study, including younger ones, information was an important factor in preventing stress, even more so than supportive care. It would not be a difficult task to prepare a simple leaflet for each operation or treatment, as well as a more general one for use particularly in non-elective admissions, giving the above details. There are now a number of well-produced books on hospital for children. Generally, any book about hospital intended for children should stimulate questions and comment from children, help them to see that their fears and reactions are normal, and also encourage them to see the experience in a positive light after discharge from hospital. Stories should be well told, with appealing illustrations, and at the same time they should give a balanced, accurate picture of life in hospital.

Pre-admission visits

Many hospitals invite children due to be admitted to hospital to visit the ward before admission and indeed the Department of Health (1996) tells parents that they can expect to see the children's ward if they want, prior to admission. Some hospitals have made videos to show to children, others take children around the ward and organize play activities intended to familiarize children with equipment routinely used in hospital. The value of such schemes has been investigated in several studies although most are very small scale. Marriner (1988), for example, introduced pre-admission visits three days prior to the scheduled admission date and evaluated the effectiveness of visits by comparing the behaviour of these children with other children who had not had a visit. The children who visited were shown around the ward and allowed to handle various pieces of equipment. Results showed that the children who had made pre-admission visits appeared to be less anxious both pre- and post-operatively and resumed usual activities quicker than children who had not. Kiely (1989), in her study of pre-admission preparation in six hospitals, evaluated the quality of visits by interviewing 80 parents whose children were in hospital. Analysis of information about pre-admission visits led Kiely to comment that the standard of these visits was variable. She also found that although four out of the six hospitals offered visits only 11 per cent of children surveyed had had a visit.

Gaughan and Sweeney (1997) evaluated a pre-admission programme for children due to be admitted to a tertiary specialist centre. They found that anxiety in relation to practical issues decreased, although anxiety in relation to medical outcomes actually increased. They concluded that this may be because families 'stopped worrying about minor practical issues and focused on the more important issue – their child' (p. 23).

The value of introducing pre-admission visits cannot be overestimated. However, from reading the research it must be said that such visits should be carefully organized and fully evaluated by the nurses involved. Robertson and Robertson (1989) pay particular attention to the timing of preparation, warning that if attempts are made to prepare children too early they can make them over-anxious. It is also very difficult to control what children will see during their visits or how they will interpret the information given. Robertson and Robertson wrote (on p. 231):

> *without the intimate knowledge that the parents have, there is a risk that, however well intentioned, the nurse or play specialist may make bad mistakes. Preparing the child is much more than giving information.*

Television

Rodin (1983), after reviewing studies on the influence of television on children, concludes that programme makers primarily use medical programmes for health education rather than hospital preparation. She feels that this is a wasted opportunity and that television could be a major source of organized preparation for children. Eiser and Patterson (1984) found that most of the children in their study had learned about hospitals through watching television but information obtained in this way is at best haphazard and at worst downright frightening. Controlling the media is beyond the reach of most nursing staff, but it is worth considering that child patients may be under some misapprehensions as a result of watching hospital programmes on television.

Play

Most studies on preparation use play as the medium for transferring information. Save the Children (1989) provides a list of the benefits of planned play programmes and a summary of this is outlined in Table 8.1 where it can be seen that the benefits of play in hospital are not restricted to preparation, but also bring an aspect of normality back into a child's life and may help them cope with things that have happened. There are a number of useful publications describing specific play

Table 8.1

Benefits of planned play programmes in hospital. Adapted from Hospital: a Deprived Environment for Children? The Case for Hospital Playschemes *(Save the Children, 1989).*

1. Play provides a normalizing experience in a stressful environment.
2. Play can prevent developmental regression.
3. Play can promote normal development and the meeting of specific developmental goals.
4. Play can reduce stress and anxiety for both the children and parents.
5. Play can facilitate communication between staff and children.
6. Play may aid diagnosis, improve recovery rates and encourage children's cooperation with hospital procedures.

programmes, and the reader is referred particularly to Petrillo and Sanger (1980) who devote a chapter to preparing children and parents for diagnostic and surgical procedures, and teaching about illness. Procedures covered include tonsillectomy, herniorrhaphy, eye surgery, closed kidney biopsy, urological surgery, cardiac catheterization and surgery, brain surgery, amputation and leukaemia. Smallwood (1988) describes the use of dolls and puppets to demonstrate medical procedures such as venepuncture, electrocardiogram and anaesthesia. Rodin (1983) designed specific preparation material in the form of games for use by children (and their parents) undergoing venepuncture, and suggests that the range of this type of material could be extended to include other medical procedures such as admission, suturing, application or removal of plaster casts, intravenous pyelograms and electro-encephalographic investigations. Rogers (1996) describes the use of educational tools including soft bodied dolls which were adapted by sewing on a felt bladder and kidneys to the doll's tummy to help children understand the working of the urinary system.

Play preparation does not necessarily require elaborate organization. Hospital dressing-up clothes and equipment can be a part of the play provision on wards (see Chapter 9) so that children can dress up and enact events that are about to happen, or have happened. It should be remembered, however, that provision of play objects is not always enough to stimulate play and it is best to have a trusted adult nearby to correct misinterpretations and answer questions, as well as to note the sorts of things that seem to be worrying children.

Emergency admissions

When children are admitted to hospital for emergency treatment, there will have been no time for specific prior preparation. Accident and emergency departments are often a child's first experience of hospital, and unfortunately some of these departments are not equipped for young children and their families. Making the accident and emergency department child friendly need not be expensive (Audit Commission, 1993) and there should at least be a separate waiting area and treatment room (Department of Health, 1996). If the environment cannot immediately be made more welcoming for children, nursing staff can still help children and parents cope with the often frightening and disorienting experience of sudden and unexpected admission to hospital by explaining in simple terms what is happening. Care should be family centred and parents can be helped to provide care even while the child is still in the Accident and Emergency department. Children should be seen immediately and have their treatment needs assessed. If they require admission they should be given a bed within two hours (Department of Health, 1996). In addition, Crocker (1980) stresses that children and their families need to be able to talk about emergency visits, about what happened and why it happened and how people felt. She calls this a debriefing and feels that it is an essential part of emergency treatment (p. 98):

Perhaps preparation and/or debriefing sessions are systematic ways of saying 'We care, we are here to help'.

This is highlighted by Miller (1996) with parents whose children were admitted following febrile convulsions. One of the most difficult aspects was when parents tried to align their own extreme fear with the calmness, coolness and casual attitude of health care professionals. Febrile convulsions might be an everyday occurrence to health care professionals, but all the parents in this small study had felt that their children were dying. One parent said (p. 31):

They said it was harmless, but if harmless means going navy blue and rigid and stopping breathing and putting on the appearance of a dead person then it is completely the wrong word to use.

The parents in this study suffered real fear and anxiety as well as guilt following the emergency admission of their children.

In practice ➤

- Hospitalization, and all that it entails, has the potential for being very frightening for children and their parents. It is important to remember that there are no events in hospital which are routine to a child or parent who has not been inside a hospital before.
- Nurses are very busy and sometimes there will be more important priorities than preparation. However, preparation does not need to be elaborate, and research shows that information alone, pitched at the right level and presented in a sensitive way, is very effective in reducing the distress of young patients and their parents.
- Most health care professionals feel that parents are the ideal people to prepare their children for hospitalization. In order to do this, however, they need to be fully informed. In addition, they need to feel welcomed and comfortable in hospital, and there may be a need for staff to emphasize to them the importance and usefulness of parents' specialized knowledge about their own children.
- Many parents and children do not ask questions because they perceive the staff as too busy. It appears from various studies that it is important that information is provided even when it is not requested. When nursing staff make the first move, the way is then opened for discussion of the concerns of individual children and their parents, and nurses can correct any misinterpretations which may have occurred.
- Since the children and parents absorb information about hospital from television programmes, schools and playgroups and from their friends and relatives, it is a good idea in any preparation to find out what they think will happen and work from there.
- The age of the child is a particularly important consideration, since children worry about different aspects of hospital at

different stages of development (see Chapter 4). Familiarity with these stages is a very useful forerunner to any decision on the content of preparation.

- Emergency admissions need special sensitivity, particularly since the environment is sometimes not suitable for children. Children and parents may need to talk about the experience with nursing staff after the crisis has passed.
- The familiarity of nursing staff with hospitals is a tremendous disadvantage to them when trying to prepare children and parents. Although very hard to do, a great effort needs to be made by staff to put themselves in the position of a patient. Look around the environment with fresh eyes and watch what children and parents are looking at. It is best never to assume that they know what things are and what will happen.

REFERENCES

Audit Commission (1993) *Children First*, Audit Commission, London.

Azarnoff, P. and Woody, P.D. (1981) Preparation of children for hospitalization in acute care hospitals in the United States. *Pediatrics*, 68, 361–8.

Ball, M., Glasper, A. and Yerrell, P. (1988) How well do we perform? Parents' perceptions of paediatric care. *The Professional Nurse*, 4(3), 115–18.

Becker, R.D.C. (1980) Psychological considerations of illness in hospitalization in childhood. *Public Health Reviews*, 9, 1–2; 9–36.

Consumers' Association (1980) *Children in Hospital*, Consumers' Association, London.

Consumers' Association (1985) *Children in Hospital*, Consumers' Association, London.

Court, S.D.M. (1976) *Fit for the Future: Report of the Committee on Child Health Services. Volumes I and II*, HMSO, London.

Crocker, E. (1980) Reactions of children to health care encounters, in *The Hospital Care of Children: A Review of Contemporary Issues* (eds G.C. Robinson and H.F. Clark), Oxford University Press, New York.

Department of Health (1996) *NHS: The Patient's Charter – Services for Children and Young People*, Department of Health, London.

Eden, O.B., Black, I., Mackinlay, C.A. and Emery, A.E.H. (1994) Communicating with Parents of Children with Cancer. *Palliative Medicine*, 8, 105–14.

Eiser, C. (1984) Communicating with sick and hospitalized children. *Journal of Child Psychology and Psychiatry*, 25, 181–9.

Eiser, C. and Patterson, D. (1984) Children's perceptions of hospital: a preliminary study. *International Journal of Nursing Studies*, 21, 45–50.

Fradd, E. (1996) The Importance of Negotiating a Care Plan. *Paediatric Nursing*, 8(6), 6–9.

Gaughan, M. and Sweeney, E. (1997) Taking Heart: Setting up a pre-admission day. *Paediatric Nursing*, 9(1), 22–3.

Glen, S.A. (1982) Hospital admission through the parents' eyes. *Nursing Times* 78(31), 1321–3.

Goodman, S. and Adams, C. (1989) 'Uncumphtable'. *Nursing Times*, 85(49), 28–31.

Harris, P.J. (1979) *Children, Their Parents and Hospital*, Unpublished PhD thesis, University of Nottingham.

Harris, P.J. (1981a) Preparation of parents and their children for a planned hospital admission. *Nursing Times*, 77(41), 1744–6.

Harris, P.J. (1981b) How parents feel. *Nursing Times*, 77(42), 1803–4.

Hawthorn, P. (1974) *Nurse, I want my mummy*! Royal College of Nursing, London.

Jolly, J. (1981) *The Other Side of Paediatrics*, Macmillan, London.

Kanneh, A. (1990) The need to communicate. *Nursing Standard*, 5(5), 19–20.

Kiely, T. (1989) Preparing children for admission to hospital. *Nursing*, Series 3(33), 42–4.

Kristjansdottir, G. (1991) Needs of Parents of Hospitalized Children. *Issues in Comprehensive Pediatric Nursing*, 14(1), 49–64.

Ley, P. (1988) *Communicating with Patients*, Croom Helm, London.

Marriner, J. (1988) A children's tour. *Nursing Times*, 84(40), 39–40.

Miller, R. (1996) The Effects on Parents of Febrile Convulsions. *Paediatric Nursing* 8(9), 28–33.

Miron, J. (1990) What children think about hospitals. *The Canadian Nurse*, 86(3), 23–5.

National Association for the Welfare of Children in Hospital (1990) Needs and services, in Children in Surgery. *Nursing Standard Special Supplement*, 4(24), 14.

Petrillo, M. and Sanger, S. (1980) *Emotional Care of Hospitalized Children: An Environmental Approach*, 2nd edn, J.B. Lippincott, Philadelphia.

Platt, H. (1959) *The Welfare of Children in Hospital. Report of the Committee on Child Health Services*, HSMO, London.

Price, B. (1988) What are nurses like? *Nursing Times*, 84(1), 42–3.

Robertson, J. and Robertson, J. (1989) *Separation and the Very Young*, Free Association Books, London.

Rodin, J. (1983) *Will This Hurt?* RCN, London.

Rogers, J. (1996) Cognitive Bladder Training in the Community. *Paediatric Nursing*, 8(8), 18–20.

Save the Children (1989) *Hospital: a Deprived Environment for Children? The Case for Hospital Playschemes*, Save the Children, London.

Smallwood, S. (1988) Preparing children for surgery. *AORN Journal*, 47(1), 177–85.

Visintainer, M.A. and Wolfer, J.A. (1975) Psychological preparation for surgical pediatric patients: the effect on children's and parents' stress responses and adjustment. *Pediatrics*, 56, 187–202.

Wattley, L.A. and Müller, D.J. (1984) *Investigating Psychology: A Practical Approach for Nursing*, Harper & Row, London.

FURTHER READING

Rodin, J. (1983) *Will This Hurt?* RCN, London.
This little book is a must for anyone thinking of designing their own preparation material, since it describes in great detail Rodin's own hard work as she set about providing preparation material for children undergoing venepuncture. The topic is expertly introduced with a review of many studies on children in hospital, providing a sound rationale for the later chapters.

Save the Children (1989) *Hospital: a Deprived Environment for Children? The Case for Hospital Playschemes*, Save the Children, London.

KEEPING HOSPITALIZED CHILDREN HAPPY 9

We have discussed the effects hospitalization has on a child, and also looked at ways of preparing children and parents for a hospital stay. We now turn to the effects there are on families over events in the hospital itself. Although happiness is a vague concept and difficult to measure, the prevention of unhappiness is very often a simple matter, requiring just a little time, thought and appreciation of what it feels like for a family facing the experience of hospitalization. The thorough preparation of families can make life in hospital happier, both for families and for staff. However, Eiser (1987) stresses that most of this preparation is aimed at children being admitted for routine surgery. Children with chronic illness and those admitted as emergencies miss out on this preparation. It is also clear that pre-admission leaflets, visits and videos cannot prepare every child and family for every aspect of hospital. Ill children and their parents may require help at each step as they pass through their stay in hospital. Paying lip-service to the concept of preparation could be a disadvantage if it was then assumed that a prepared family could then cope satisfactorily without further assistance.

Much attention has been directed at finding ways in which the experience of hospital could be made less stressful for young children. Poster (1983) categorized the possible approaches according to their aims.

1. Those approaches that are intended to decrease the exposure to the stress of hospitalization, and include outpatient care, day surgery and reduced separation through unrestricted visiting by parents and siblings.
2. Those approaches that increase families' ability to cope in hospital, namely in hospital preparation for surgery, tests and procedures, play and discussion programmes, parent education and involvement in care, and lastly, encouraging young children to bring into hospital their special objects such as blankets or their favourite toys.
3. Those approaches that provide external resources such as increased availability of support groups for parents of hospitalized children, increased availability of literature and films on hospital, counselling during and after hospital, and emotional support for nursing staff.

It is clear that there are many factors which affect a child's experience of hospital, either positively or negatively, but here we concern ourselves with those that impinge on the hospital stay itself, that is, those falling into Poster's second category. These include hospital routines and treatments, aspects of the hospital environment, play and education while in hospital, staff organization, the presence of other people with the child and, to conclude, the special considerations of accident and emergency departments.

HOSPITAL ROUTINES AND TREATMENT PROCEDURES

Many hospital routines are carried out for traditional reasons, rather than anything else. Therefore, any alterations in these routines, while resulting in no less efficiency or greater effort, could change for the better the experience of children and their parents in hospital.

Admission and Planning Care

In an article entitled *Hospital admission through the parents' eyes*, Glen (1982), a ward sister, discusses a theme mentioned in Chapter 8, that is, that when preparing children and parents, a nurse's familiarity with hospitals is a disadvantage. She suggests that sensitivity is particularly required when admitting a child:

> *The admission procedure should never be considered as a routine nursing ritual. The admission procedure is the child and her parents' first contact with the ward, and their first impression can greatly influence their subsequent experience.*

Fradd (1996) further elaborates this point and stresses the importance of early negotiation between the nurse and the family in relation to care planning. This, Fradd suggests, helps in terms of the cooperation of all parties, the understanding of the child and family about the care and nurses' understanding of the patient's wishes. This process takes time and is an activity which requires skill and sensitivity. Parents need time to question at the assessment stage, and staff should try and understand this need and answer all questions instead of labelling the parents as being difficult, or awkward, and avoiding them. The initial assessment provides opportunity to get to know the child and family and provides familiar ground for later interactions such as the name by which the child is known, names and ages of siblings, what 'granny' is called, information on favourite toys, what the child says if a toilet is needed, food preferences, play preferences, favourite activities, and names of pets. In this way the child is treated first as a person and second as a patient, and this is as important to children as it is to adults.

A number of children in one study (Harris, 1981a) were said by their parents to have benefited from the researcher's presence, simply because she asked them questions about themselves. The mother of a 9 year old boy said:

> *He felt it was nice to have someone who was interested in him as a person, his thoughts and feelings were important, he wasn't just a patient.*

Many of the parents in Harris's (1981a) study also felt reassured because the researcher knew their children and their preferences (from a brief home interview during the week before admission) and had asked questions similar to those mentioned above. It does seem to be important to parents that their children's individuality is recognized, and such information should be incorporated into the care plan and should be readily available.

Another important area of concern relating to the admission procedure is the need for nurses to be both sensitive and perceptive to each situation. Williamson and Williamson (1987) describe the admission of their daughter, Elizabeth, by a student nurse who asked questions without explaining why the information was needed. Robbins (1987) makes reference to the admission of Elizabeth and asks why a qualified children's nurse was not available who could have 'modified the admission process to suit the occasion'. We again appreciate that staff shortages may make it difficult for qualified nurses always to admit children. However, the first impressions of the child and family will lay the foundation for the rest of the child's stay in hospital and care taken early on may prevent excessive stress which will eventually involve nursing time later on. On a similar note, Swanwick (1996) emphasizes the importance of being aware of the cultural needs of children and their families. We live in a multicultural society and knowledge of cultural needs can prevent the 'unintentional blunder' which can be distressing for both the family and the nurse.

The admission procedure very often involves a substantial waiting time. The Consumers' Association survey (1980) found that only 54 per cent of children whose admissions were planned went directly to their wards, 24 per cent went to reception and 16 per cent went to an admission room. Children who did not go directly to their wards were understandably irritated by the admission system in one particular hospital, which often involved a long wait of up to three hours outside the ward. In a number of cases they felt that this lowered a child's confidence. It was suggested that the waiting time, if inevitable, could be used in a more constructive way and could be arranged in more pleasant surroundings than a dark hospital corridor. For example, specific hospital routines could be demonstrated and other preparation for particular operations be given during the afternoon of admission. The provision of information could be an important feature of the admission procedure; parents could also take advantage of this time by having a trained member of staff available to answer their questions. Suggestions such as this may evoke a hollow laugh in readers at this point, since staff shortages mean that those staff available are involved in essential tasks. However, it is worth considering whether these tasks are all necessary; perhaps, given the importance of information-giving, staff time could be rearranged according to different priorities.

As a final point on admission, some of the children in Harris's (1979) study ended up near other children who were vomiting in reaction to an anaesthetic received earlier in the day. There was an immediate change in the admitted children's attitude from cheerful anticipation to apprehension. One boy shook and turned away, then cried inconsolably. His father also found this most distasteful and had to leave. Two of the admitted children, previously quite happy, cried to go home. A little thought and reorganization could have prevented this unfortunate start to these children's hospital stay.

The physical examination

An inevitable part of a hospital stay is the physical examination. Moss (1981), an assistant professor at an American college of nursing, discusses the special problems inherent in examining young children. Before 2 years of age, the level of a child's cooperation mainly depends on temperament, fatigue level and the skills of the practitioner in providing distraction, whereas older children can actively cooperate (or actively not cooperate). Moss points out that the fear arising from painful procedures (e.g. injections, finger pricks) may be transferred to the normally painless physical examination and cause a child to struggle. The physical findings obtained from a cooperative child are clearly likely to be more accurate and complete than those from one who has screamed and fought through the whole examination. As Moss emphasizes:

> *It is in the best interests of the pediatric nurse practitioner to have a compliant child, even though a few more minutes may be spent with him initially.*

Robinson and Collier (1997) also studied the issue of procedures by surveying 394 paediatric nurses about restraining children during procedures. They concluded that most nurses felt that it was the restraint rather than pain which was the most likely cause of distress. Parental presence was felt to be desirable and issues such as the legal position regarding restraint and consent was raised. Moss (1981) also raised this point and emphasized that she always asks the children if they would prefer to be examined on a parent's lap or on the examination table, and she encourages children to put their hands on the diaphragm of the stethoscope and tell her when it is warm enough to place on the chest. Measures like these give children a little bit of choice and control in an environment in which they can otherwise feel very powerless. Moss's account of the best way to give a full physical examination is not reported in full here, since generally it is doctors who carry out this procedure in British hospitals, but interested readers are referred to her informative article.

Specific treatment procedures

One of the most important prerequisites for a successful treatment procedure is to explain what is being done. Most good textbooks on paediatric nursing (e.g. Foster *et al.*, 1989) give specific suggestions on how to demonstrate equipment to children before using it on them.

Most suggest allowing the child to hold and play with safe equipment such as flashlights, stethoscopes and tongue blades, and demonstrating these on a doll, the parent, or a member of staff. Carter (1994) suggests a number of useful strategies which are helpful when the child is undergoing short-duration painful procedures, including distraction, relaxation, hypnosis and imagery. Information, preparation and the development of coping strategies are, according to Carter, 'key elements in reducing the pain and distress associated with procedural pain' (p. 113). Carter states that one of the most stressful events is an injection, and refers to a number of studies supporting this view. She adds that steps must be taken to avoid intramuscular injections which are 'the worst hurt' (p. 60) for children. Similar procedures such as fingerpricks, blood tests, spinal taps and intravenous infusions are also found particularly stressful.

Children also need time to 'debrief' after a painful procedure, and staff should talk to them about their experiences. Just because a needle has been removed does not mean that the injection site is no longer painful. Children also need positive reinforcement, such as telling them that they were very brave.

Another procedure with frightening features similar to injections is suturing. Beckemeyer and Bahr (1980) describe a typical scene where a 5 year old's wound is to be sutured:

> *As soon as the nurse injects a local anaesthetic into his wound the child's fears of forthcoming horror are confirmed. A severe burning sensation follows and by the time the anaesthetic takes effect, the child is generally so frightened and convinced that he will be hurt again that he interprets all sensations as painful.*

The authors then describe the same type of situation, but this time the nurse used a special technique:

> *While shielding the needle from the child's view with one hand the nurse slowly dripped some anaesthetic into the open wound taking several minutes to do this. After the anaesthetic had taken partial effect, she injected the rest, all the while keeping the needle hidden by her hand.*

Beckemeyer and Bahr (1980) found many articles on suturing lacerations, which instructed that the wound be properly, surgically anaesthetized or that it be anaesthetized by inserting the needle under the skin edges, and they comment: 'Incredibly, these articles seemed to be dealing with a wound, not a person'. They did, however, find a number of articles giving sound evidence for the efficacy of the method described above, and suggest that it is not more widely used because staff feel it is more time consuming. Yet the only time involved is in the topical application of the anaesthetic, which produces sufficient numbing for the introduction of the needle through the anaesthetized area without pain.

As with the physical examination, the physical effect will be better if the child is happier, suturing will be easier and more successful.

Going to the operating department

One of the most frequently discussed issues concerning the care of children in hospital is the presence of parents in the anaesthetic room. Whilst it is a much more usual occurrence, and the Department of Health (1996) tells parents that, where circumstances permit, they have the right to be with the child, it is an issue which is still debated probably because the induction of anaesthesia can be particularly traumatic for both the child and family and both can become extremely distressed (Perthen, 1990). Perthen in her study of anaesthetists tried to ascertain why parents were not routinely permitted to accompany their children in the anaesthetic room. The reasons noted by Perthen were:

1. local custom: operating department rules and regulations;
2. fear of increased risk of infection;
3. problem of coping with two potential patients (parents may require attention, especially if they faint);
4. training experience may be hampered by parental presence; and
5. fear of having a potential critic in the anaesthetic room.

Perthen also carried out a small study to find out if the anaesthetists' fears about the potential disruption caused by having parents present during induction of anaesthesia were accurate. She found that far from being disruptive, the children derived benefit from the presence of a parent and induction was able to take place in a 'relaxed atmosphere'. These findings were supported by Coulson (1988) in a study of 32 children who were accompanied by a parent to the anaesthetic room. This author concluded that:

> *anxieties about critical or hysterical parents who may cause complications are unfounded ... generally parents should be actively encouraged to accompany their child in the anaesthetic room, and be given guidance on what they can do to help.*

Clearly, the advantages for the majority of children of having a parent present during the potentially traumatic experience of induction of anaesthesia must outweigh the possible disadvantages of the rare occasion when a parent becomes unduly distressed.

Little things mean a lot

In Harris's research (1979) it was often found that a small action on the part of the staff while carrying out routine procedures was often much appreciated by the children. For example, fastening a name tag to a child's doll or treating a bump on teddy's head with sticking plaster after having fallen out of bed, can make a surprising difference to a child's overall attitude to hospital. A number of children, in answer to the question 'What did you like best about hospital?', mentioned that they liked the ride on the trolley down to the theatre. All were in the tonsil-lectomy ward where a number of children were put on the trolley together, teddies included, and transported down in the lift, often with much laughing and kicking in spite of the premedication. None of the children in the other ward enjoyed their ride to the theatre, perhaps because they went down one at a time in more sober circumstances. An opportunity was therefore wasted to put a bit of fun into the hospital experience. Also on the subject of trolleys, Fradd (1986) describes how the nurses in her hospital have disguised the traditional trolleys to look like Thomas the Tank Engine. Jolly (1981) describes one hospital that capitalizes on children's love of badges – of any sort. Ordinary cardboard labels with safety pins on the back are used as badges identifying children on diets, to those having operations, or who needs fluids to be measured or collected. (Whilst we endorse this practice for the purposes cited here, the practice of writing a diagnosis (e.g. diabetic) on a badge is unaccep-table. It not only labels the child but also breaches the child's right to confidentiality.) Ainsworth (1987) discusses the use of limited edition designer hats for children who had their heads shaved for neurosurgery.

Attention to how a child perceives a situation can be very rewarding to staff. Jolly (1981) points out that children are often reluctant to go to a different part of the hospital for tests, treatment or to play in case their parents will not be able to find them. She suggests leaving a large note on the child's bed 'Mummy, Johnny has gone to x-ray. Back by 12 o'clock'. Jolly (1988) comments on the practice of bed-moving and suggests that children find this disturbing and fear their families won't be able to find them. Harris (1979) also found children became upset when it was necessary to move their beds to a different ward at night for reasons of staff economy. It was not routinely explained to children that their parents would be told exactly where they were, or that they would be back in their rightful place by the next morning. Children also became upset by the routine distribution of postoperative equipment (such as vomit bowls) on the morning of the operation. Again, very little effort is required to delay this until after the children have gone down to the operating theatre.

Jolly (1981) discusses another routine activity that appears unnecessary, that of waking sleeping children. She says (p. 120) there is no need for this, except to administer medication:

I know of no good reason for them to be bathed, dressed and fed before the day staff arrive.

The message keeps coming through; treat a child as a person. In this context a child's need for privacy is very important. The Consumers' Association (1980) found that children in their survey were very sensitive to embarrassment. Just over a quarter of the hospitals never screened children, or only did this in extreme cases. Harris's study (1979) included boys and girls up to 12 years old, and some were very embarrassed by being taken to their beds on admission and told to get undressed without anyone thinking of putting screens around their bed. One 11 year old was very put out when given an operating gown that was too small. A nurse told him that she would get another, but after half an hour came back to say she could not find another one. He kept asking if he could put a blanket around him to go to the toilet, but a nurse said she would bring a bedpan instead, which made him more embarrassed since he was being teased by younger children in the ward already. Just a little understanding is required, particularly on those occasions where a child, long since toilet trained, wets the bed. Weller (1980) stresses that in this situation nurses need to take great care to reassure child and parents that this is a temporary situation which will pass, and not indicate any displeasure by tone of voice or attitude, as the child will already be very distressed at his or her incontinence. Although it may be very hard for nurses to see familiar ward routines with new eyes, let alone through a child's eyes, the research quoted here suggests that it is certainly well worth the effort.

Food

The Consumers' Association (1980) found that all the children in their survey loudly criticized hospital food. A psychologist, advising the Association, commented that all children may be expected to have fads and are prone to criticize institutional food, but adds that the food may have acted as a symbol for wider criticism which they felt unable to verbalize. Whatever the reasons behind the criticism, sensitivity and understanding on the part of the staff will help. Jolly (1981) points out that children are not usually used to a cooked breakfast, and that plated meals are unsatisfactory since children tend to eat the pudding first. Fradd (1986) tackled the criticisms of food by children by closely liaising with catering staff and inviting the cooks to the wards to discuss with the children what they wanted. Careful management of drinks and mealtimes in hospital can provide a routine that is nearer the child's home experience, and thus reduce the discontinuity between home and hospital. Care must also be taken to ensure that children who are on special diets, whether for medical or cultural reasons, are not made to feel stigmatized in any way.

HOSPITAL ENVIRONMENT

The importance of the setting in which the care of children takes place has been highlighted frequently in the literature. NAWCH (1988) in their *Quality Checklist No. 6* state:

> *Children should be in an environment furnished and equipped to meet their requirements and which conforms to recognized standards of safety and supervision. The design and facilities of the children's ward should be attractive and welcoming, purpose built and adapted for the use of children.*

In their *Quality Review* (NAWCH 1989) they elaborate (on Page 20):

> *Distress affects the child's recovery and so it is important to understand how a child sees the hospital. Comfortable child-oriented surroundings help to lower children's anxiety and make them more cooperative with staff. The ward or clinic should provide opportunities for activity, play and social exchange.*

Fradd (1986) suggests that making the ward environment as much like home as possible will have an effect on the 'success of any child's stay'. Surroundings should be attractive and bright and age appropriate. Fradd emphasizes that adolescents, for example, need a dayroom rather than a playroom and the Audit Commission (1993) suggest that they should have access to kitchen facilities. Rodin (1983) adds that a welcoming environment also helps parents to attend to instructions and explanations, to treat a child with more patience and understanding, and to accept distressing diagnoses with greater calm.

Addressing the question of a child-centred environment, the *Standards of Care* Project (RCN, 1990) emphasizes the importance of safety in *Standard 5*. Attention should be given to the equipment, toys and the level of supervision. A knowledge of child development will help nurses to identify age-appropriate toys and games and will also give nurses knowledge about children's capabilities. A 3 year old, for example, may have no hesitation about walking out of the ward to find his absent mother.

Other studies have identified aspects of hospital that bother children and many of the points highlighted could be changed without too much time or cost. A study by Goodman and Adams (1989), for example, showed that the hospital smell was the thing that children mentioned most frequently. It would be relatively simple to abolish such smells with the use of air freshener. Other hospitals have made unusual efforts to entertain children who visit them. In the USA, the Boston Floating Hospital has large squares of plasterboard (graffiti boards) above the beds, which are repainted whenever the room is decorated. In between the painting, they carry remarks from one patient to the next (Hardgrove and Dawson, 1972):

> *Harry was here but now he's gone, left his appendix to carry on.*
> *Mary went home but never mind, her adenoids got left behind.*

The environment can have a great effect on encouraging, or discouraging communication between staff and parents, children and other children, parents and other parents and between parents and child. Conversations with other children were of great importance to the children in Harris's (1979) study, and although they often managed to carry these out around each other's beds, a room adjoining the ward, preferably with a television, would have been much appreciated for the purpose of social activities. Many children like to watch television together; certain television programmes are a normal part of life for many children and provide a useful link with home while they are in hospital. It was not only children who would have appreciated a room away from their beds where they could relax, converse and enjoy their leisure in a more familiar way. Many parents would also have liked somewhere they could go to relax during a long day of story reading, talking and playing with their child, a room providing a telephone, facilities to make drinks, chat to other parents, or feed a baby.

Finally, a letter from a mother to a newsletter (NAWCH, 1984a) shows the effect the environment can have on a child. She describes two hospitals in which her son David had stitches in his head. In the first the furniture and staff were arranged in such a way that she could stand next to the bed on the opposite side to the staff while David received his stitches. In the second hospital, not only was she discouraged from entering, and told that if she insisted on coming in she would have to sit over in the corner, but the arrangements of bed, instrument trolley and staff meant there was nowhere else for her to be except in the corner, away from her child.

PLAY

Why is play important in hospital? What sort of conditions are likely to encourage the children to play and to get the most out of their play? What sort of equipment is needed? These are the sorts of questions which nurses may ask when considering specifically how to keep children happy on a paediatric ward and this section looks at some of the work that has been done on play in a hospital setting.

Functions of play in hospital

In Chapter 8, we discussed the benefits of play in hospital. These include the maintenance of normal activities, which reduces both the strangeness of the environment and the discontinuity between home and hospital; expression of concern, confusions and fear through play; reduction of incidents and injuries by provision of a safe outlet for energies; 'playing hospitals' to reduce fear of instruments and treatments; and providing an antidote for boredom. There are many theories about and definitions of play, but Crocker (1980) stresses that most of these are not broad enough to explain all the different types and contexts of play. She suggests that play may be accepted to mean those activities that involve a child in exploring, investigating, manipulating and problem-solving, including role-playing and repeating (or reliving) events.

Poster (1983) emphasizes that play is a natural activity which allows children to learn and experiment with the things around them; it is also an activity in which the child has control, can decide what happens and when, and can become more efficient at doing things. A review of research on play in hospital leads Bolig (1984) to conclude that there appear to be four main functions.

1. to provide diversion, that is some kind of simple occupation to take children's minds off what is going on around them;
2. 'playing out' problems and anxieties;
3. restoring normal aspects of life; and
4. aiding understanding so that, through play, a child can become more aware of hospital events and can communicate fears.

Conditions for play

Play is clearly important to a child in hospital, and in many hospitals it is intended to serve multiple functions. However, encouraging play in hospital is not the same as encouraging play in, say, a playgroup or in the home. Bolig (1984) notes that any brief and intense stress such as a smack, may render normally functioning children 'playless'. The physiological and psychological stresses of illness and hospitalization can make it very difficult for a child to play in the normal way as she notes (p. 323):

> *In the absence of familiar persons, objects and routines and with the real or perceived threat of injections, medications and procedures, many children while hospitalized cannot spontaneously play.*

Bolig emphasizes the need for a child-orientated atmosphere, with appropriate toys and creative materials and the presence of a trusted, permission-giving and responsive adult. In the absence of such a person, most young children cannot play and even older children need the presence of such an adult at least initially until they make friends.

Some convincing results were obtained in a very early study by Harvey (1966) who found that when supervised play was provided, children engaged in 'settled activities' for an average of 39.4 minutes, whereas in the absence of the play specialist children engaged in such activities for an average of only 3.8 minutes.

Does this mean that wards without a play specialist can never provide ideal conditions for play? Not if Crocker's (1980) advice is heeded. She emphasizes that even in places where play staff exist, it should not be assumed that they are the only 'players'; all staff who come into contact with children should see themselves as 'play opportunists', ready and able to stimulate and react to children's play needs. Crocker recommends some healthy 'role-blurring' rather than professional 'territoriality'. Bolig (1984) notes that parents too have an important function here, but they very often change their behaviour towards their children once the children are hospitalized. They are uncertain what they can and cannot do with, or for, their children, and may assume a sickroom role, quiet, soothing and reassuring. In such cases, it is helpful if staff can provide the necessary information and encouragement for parents to resume a more normal playful relationship with their children, to the benefit of themselves, their children and the staff who are caring for their children.

Play equipment

Environments (cheerful, child-orientated) and attitudes (flexible, encouraging, accepting) are as important, if not more important than equipment, but a number of publications exist which give plenty of ideas for hospital play equipment. Weller's (1980) book is devoted entirely to play in hospital, and Action for Sick Children publish a number of leaflets such as *Messy Play in Hospital* which list useful equipment. The reader is referred to these for the detail they provide, but in general the needs of children in terms of actual play equipment are not great. Crocker (1980) suggests that a toy doctor's bag, some teddy bear and doll patients and hospital clothing should be around at all times. She describes one hospital which has developed some life-sized puppets that can demonstrate the visual side of various surgical and medical procedures; for example the neurosurgery puppet's hair is removable in sections; the intensive care unit puppet is a dog who encourages children to do deep breathing postoperatively (she does not say how), the ear, nose and throat puppet's tonsils actually come out, the general surgery puppet has a chest scar from open heart surgery and has monitor leads attached to the chest.

Equipment does not of course have to be this elaborate, although miniature uniforms are usually appreciated in which children can dress up and enact the events that have happened or are about to happen. Rodin (1983) recommends hospital dressing-up clothes for their therapeutic value and also to give staff clues as to how much the children understand. The play can often reveal unnecessary fears, such as of death or amputation, which might arise out of the child's knowledge of the hospital experiences of relatives, or fears resulting merely from the child's immaturity, such as that any blood taken needs to be replaced immediately.

Space does not permit a detailed account of play equipment here. If you have the opportunity to develop play and play materials in your children's ward, you will find some useful books in the Further Reading section.

EDUCATION IN HOSPITAL

In many ways the functions of education in hospital are similar to those of play. Crocker (1980) suggests:

1. going to school is a normal activity and, as such, can help reduce the strangeness of a hospital;
2. schoolwork and related activities give children chances to succeed and show what they can do; and
3. doing school work can mean to many children 'you will be going home; it is important to keep up with your classmates', thereby shifting the emphasis from the actual hospital stay to the return home and life being normal again.

The Quality Review (NAWCH, 1989) describes the job of a hospital teacher and outlines that whilst, because of shorter hospital stays, the educational value for the child in hospital is minimal school provides a means of allaying anxiety and provides a link between their normal lives and hospital. For longer stay children the role of the teacher involves close liaison with the child's normal school so that the child can continue to follow the same curriculum. The role of the teacher will also vary according to the ages and mobility of the children as well as the severity of illness.

Fradd (1986) discusses how teachers in one hospital become involved with children following neurosurgery and head injuries while they are still in intensive care. This early contact by teachers acts as a stimulus for the child and as soon as he or she is able, the child will attend the hospital school with other children. The teaching staff, according to Fradd, care for the children's intravenous infusions and drains and only under exceptional circumstances will a nurse remain with the child. Fradd writes:

> school is one of only a few normal activities we are able to encourage in an otherwise unusual and unnatural routine.

The Quality Review (NAWCH, 1989) notes that most parents do not expect teachers to be available in hospital. Education does however take up a great deal of time in the lives of children outside the hospital environment and for many children it is appropriate that it should continue during hospitalization. Some children, for example those being treated for skin disorders or having orthopaedic corrections, are not ill at all, and schooling may occupy a substantial and important proportion of their day. Education is particularly important for longer-term children who may become very institutionalized. Parents should naturally be involved in this process and Lavelle (1994) suggests that an individual programme can be worked out according to the child's capability. If the child is attending a hospital school then the cooperation of other health care professionals is needed. It is a difficult enough task for a teacher faced with perhaps 20 children of different ages and abilities, and who are constantly changing, without having to deal with constant interruptions from other staff. Nor is it beneficial for the child or other children in the class.

STAFF ORGANIZATION

In discussing the role of the children's nurse, McQuaid (1996) stresses that a child should come into contact with as few people as possible while in hospital. Harris (1981c) suggests that patient assignment would certainly have alleviated some of the problems which parents in her study felt their children faced in hospital, for example knowing no-one by name to whom they could turn in distress. Brown's (1989) study, which compared task allocation with patient assignment in two paediatric settings, also highlights the benefits of patient assignment. With task assignment, the care of any one child is necessarily fragmented and with the trend towards shorter stays for children and shorter hours for nursing staff, nurses are less likely to come to know the children as individuals. This was emphasized in Harris's (1979) study by the inability of nurses to complete a behaviour rating scale on the children for the purposes of the research. They did not feel they saw enough of them to assess their behaviour.

Brown (1989) suggests that the nurse's view of a child is fragmented because of the variety of tasks being performed, and that it is difficult for a child to attract a nurse's attention. One of the reasons is that when a nurse enters a ward it is generally because she has something to do, something *else* from the child's point of view. The Consumers' Association's (1980) survey also showed that nurses were often thought by children to be too busy to spend time with individual patients. Thus children did not feel they could interrupt nurses to attend to their small needs, talk to them or ask questions.

The 'Children's Charter' (Department of Health, 1996) recommends that each child and family should have a named nurse through whom they can channel communication. Primary nursing can also aid more open communication (Farrell, 1995) and 'generates for the nurse a sense of increased involvement with a child and family' (p. 562).

THE PRESENCE OF OTHER PEOPLE

We can now look in more detail at the subject of visiting. Having established in Chapter 8 that the presence of parents in particular is important both for the physical and psychological recovery of children, this section discusses the practicalities of the existence of other people (i.e. besides staff and patients) on a children's ward.

Parents

The presence of a parent contributes significantly to a child's successful adaptation to hospital. The NAWCH (1986) survey noted that, while many hospitals have instituted liberal visiting hours, rooming-in policies do not always reflect what is actually taking place. Parents are not always *encouraged* to stay and beds are not always available for them. Parents may be assigned Z-bed in a playroom or a chair in a ward and whilst this may be acceptable for one night parents can soon become exhausted through lack of sleep. It then becomes very tempting to leave the child for a good night's sleep at home. This practice may also be totally unacceptable for parents from some cultures. The *Quality Review* (NAWCH, 1989) set standards for parental accommodation and offers a formula for working out requirements. It also recommends that hospitals carefully monitor parental bed occupancy and the Audit Commission (1993) adds that parental satisfaction with facilities is rarely considered. Without careful audit, hospitals will not have knowledge of the children who are unaccompanied at night and hence will not have sufficient evidence to suggest making changes to improve the situation. If a parent is not resident it may mean that the child is left alone to face stressful procedures and experiences, such as injections, enemas, catheterizations and the pre- and post-operative period. Rutter (1981) warns that the circumstances experienced by a child during separation from parents can make a difference to a child's emotional response.

The report *Parents Staying Overnight in Hospital with their Children* discussed by Sadler (1988) stresses that parents should be informed of the importance to the child of their presence at night. The report also recommends that beds should be provided for one parent for every child under 5 years old, for 75 per cent of 5–7 year olds, for 50 per cent of 8–11 year olds and for 25 per cent of 12–16 year olds. As well as a bed, parents also need access to a sitting room and shower/toilet facilities (NAWCH, 1989). All facilities should be next to the child or within 'dressing gown distance'. This is important if parents are to participate fully in the care of the child and in decision-making in partnership with health care professionals.

A valuable perspective on parents is provided by Thornes (NAWCH, 1984b), who emphasizes parents are not visitors but equal partners with hospital staff. At each stage they need to be involved, to know what is wrong with their child and why treatment is being given. Casey and Mobbs (1988) have formalized partnership with parents by designing a comprehensive and workable model of nursing for use in childcare settings. The model facilitates negotiation and clarifies the roles of the child, the family and the nurse and promotes a family centred approach to care. Woodfield (1997) goes further and suggests that consideration should be given to the development of a 'parents' charter' which would be beneficial in ensuring that the needs of parents are fully met.

Brothers, sisters and friends

The Consumers' Association (1980) found in the matter of visiting that 'hospitals were particularly ambivalent about brothers and sisters and indeed children generally', yet their interviews with children suggested that great significance is attached to visits from brothers and sisters, schoolfriends, grandmothers and others. The presence of other child patients does not always mitigate this. Children sometimes find it hard to approach other patients and sometimes the disparity in ages is too great for friendships to develop. When in hospital, children need reminding about other aspects of their lives and letters from school and visits by siblings and friends are all extremely important. Children in hospital need to be kept in touch with other members of their families. Not only do sick children need to see their brothers and sisters, but the siblings themselves also need reassurance about the one in hospital, although careful preparation of siblings prior to visiting is of extreme importance. Morrison (1997), for example, found in her study that siblings actually found visiting 'anxiety inducing' (p. 27).

The lonely child

Goldsborough (NAWCH, 1984a) discusses the problem of the child whose parents rarely visit, and (on p. 2) emphasizes the child's right to a one-to-one relationship:

> *It is not a question of having* an *adult with a child, but the* same *adult.*

In spite of more liberal visiting policies there are still a number of unaccompanied children in hospital (NAWCH, 1989; Audit Commission, 1993). It is important that unvisited children are given special attention, indeed that they are *noticed*. Jolly (1981) notes that it is not always the rule that visits are recorded, so with changes of staff it may not come to light that a child has not been visited. Wherever possible, organization of staff or volunteers should ensure that such a child has some consistent and loving support.

EMERGENCY ADMISSIONS

Accidents and emergencies in children are usually managed in the main department of the hospital, where about 30 per cent of the patients are children, and where few of the nursing and medical staff have any post-registration paediatric training (Consumers' Association, 1985; NAWCH, 1989). Yet 20–25 per cent of the child population is seen annually in the accident and emergency department (NAWCH, 1989). By the age of 5 years, 44 per cent of children have had an accident requiring medical attention and this is, in many cases, their first experience of hospital. The departments are often not equipped to deal with children (Smith, 1997). The Audit Commission (1993) advocate the provision of separate treatment rooms where children should be shielded from the sights and sounds of critically injured patients; a curtained cubicle does not provide enough privacy to prevent a child from being terrified on hearing screams of pain. Often the child's injury is minor compared to the more seriously ill patients who require immediate attention and children should be assessed immediately (Department of Health, 1996; Cole, 1997). Nurses should go periodically to see paediatric patients in the waiting room just to provide a few comforting words and explanations, so that the crisis tone of the emergency room can be considerably reduced.

This suggestion, by its very simplicity, sums up much of what we have been trying to convey in this chapter. Just a little time and thought on the part of the nursing staff and a genuine attempt to put themselves in a child's or parent's precarious position can improve the experience of hospitalization for young patients and their families.

QUALITY ASSURANCE

To conclude this chapter we feel it is important to look at the issue of quality assurance in relation to the psychological care of children in hospital. Ball *et al.* (1988, p. 115) define quality assurance as:

A process of looking at a given situation and appraising it against a measure or set standard.

Throughout this section we have discussed issues relating to psychological need and, while it appears that much progress has been made in both the physical and psychological care of children, much of the research cited in this chapter shows that there is still room for improvement. Setting standards and evaluating the quality of care against those standards is an effective way of highlighting areas of weakness, agreeing targets for future practice and measuring the effectiveness of change.

NAWCH (1988) has published a set of '*quality checklists*' based on the 1984 NAWCH charter, which enable managers to compare the care offered in their hospital against the criteria identified by NAWCH. The checklists were followed up by the *Quality Review* (NAWCH, 1989). Other tools for measuring the quality of care for children are available such as *Junior Monitor* (Galvin and Goldstone, 1988). The Royal College of Nursing (1990) has also produced a broad set of standards for the care of children in hospital. These standards can be adapted for use in different settings and nurses can use the format to write more specific standards of care relating to their own area of practice.

While writing and measuring standards can be seen as yet more work for already over-stretched staff, they can provide an objective picture of what care is being given to children and families. Williams (1989) described how *Junior Monitor* results were used to the advantage of the nurses:

Analysis of Junior Monitor showed that the workload within the wards was high and that additional nursing staff were required to cope with that workload in order to deliver an improved level of care.

◄ *In practice*

- Even where families have been prepared for the hospital experience, they will still need understanding and help at each step in the hospitalization process.
- Many hospital routines are carried out more because of tradition than anything else. It is well worth nurses' efforts to look again at their actions and interactions with children and consider whether the action is really necessary; how it might look from the point of view of parents and children; and how it might be changed.
- First impressions are important in influencing parents' and children's reactions in hospital, so the admission procedure needs careful scrutiny to see how it could be made more welcoming, and how it could provide more information for both staff and families.

- Little things mean a lot. In addition to re-thinking established hospital routines, it is rewarding to add thoughtful touches, such as fastening a name tag to a child's doll. These increase children's feelings of being a person rather than a condition and add a bit of harmless fun to the whole experience.
- The actual hospital environment can also substantially affect the happiness of its users. Small changes such as pictures on the walls, bright colours, a kettle for parents, an air freshener to disguise the hospital smell, and the arrangement of furniture to encourage communication can make a big difference.
- Hospital equipment, although completely familiar to staff, can appear frightening to parents and children. It is best either to keep it out of sight, or explain what it is for.
- Play is an important part of hospitalization, for diversion, 'playing out' anxieties, restoring a sense of normality and aiding understanding. It appears best for all staff to be involved in encouraging play, rather than simply leaving everything to a play leader (where available). Parents too may need information as to how much play their ill child can take, and they may need encouragement too.
- Education is also important for maintaining some normality, for giving children a chance to show what they can do, and as reassurance that they will be going back to school, that is, going home.
- Children need as much consistent care as is possible while in hospital, and re-thinking staff organization (e.g. changing from daily patient assignment to primary nursing) can make consistent care easier to achieve.
- Viewing 'talking and listening to children' as a valid and high priority part of a nurse's role can help children a great deal, and will be much appreciated by parents and children alike.
- Parents are extremely important to children while they are in hospital, but they do not always realize this. An explanation of the importance of frequent visiting and partnership in care, and a warm welcome from staff while parents visit will be very beneficial for children. Visits from brothers, sisters and schoolfriends will also be much appreciated and help maintain the all important link with home.
- Unvisited children need extra attention, and wherever possible a one-to-one relationship with an adult while they are in hospital. If staff can keep a record of visitors, it will be apparent which children are missing out.
- Families admitted in an emergency need sensitive reassurance and frequent information, particularly if they have to wait some time in the accident and emergency department for treatment.
- Continuity with home experience appears to be very important for children. Apart from play and education, continuity can be provided by talking to children about their life outside the

hospital, brothers and sisters, friends, pets and other aspects of home life. If a list of names of relations and pets is kept at the end of the bed, anyone who sees the child has a starting point for conversations about home.

REFERENCES

Ainsworth, H. (1987) Making it happy. *Nursing Times* 83(30), 41–2.

Audit Commission (1993) *Children First*, Audit Commission, London.

Ball, M., Glasper, A. and Yerrell, P. (1988) How well do we perform? Parents' perceptions of paediatric care. *The Professional Nurse*, 4(3), 115–18.

Beckemeyer, P. and Bahr, J.E. (1980) Helping toddlers and preschoolers cope while suturing their minor lacerations. *American Journal of Maternal and Child Nursing*, 5(5; Sept/Oct), 326–30.

Bolig, R. (1984) Play in hospital settings, in *Child's Play: Developmental and Applied*, (eds T.D. Yawkey and A.D. Pellegrini), Lawrence Erlbaum, Hillsdale, NJ.

Brown, R. (1989) *Individualised Care*, Scutari Press, Middlesex.

Carter, B. (1994) *Child and Infant Pain: Principles of Nursing Care and Management*, Chapman and Hall, London.

Casey, A. and Mobbs, S. (1988) Partnership in practice. *Nursing Times*, 84(44), 67–8.

Cole, R. (1997) Triage in the Children's A and E Department. *Paediatric Nursing*, 9(2), 29–34.

Consumers' Association (1980) *Children in Hospital*, Consumers' Association, London.

Consumers' Association (1985) *Children in Hospital*, Consumers' Association, London.

Coulson, D. (1988) A proper place for parents. *Nursing Times*, 84(19), 26–8.

Crocker, E. (1980) Reactions of children to health care encounters, in *The Hospital Care of Children: A Review of Contemporary Issues*, (eds G.C. Robinson and H.F. Clark), Oxford University Press, New York.

Department of Health (1996) *NHS: The Patient's Charter – Services for Children and Young People*, Department of Health, London.

Eiser, C. (1987) What children think about hospitals and illness. *The Professional Nurse*, 3(2), 53–4.

Farrell, M. (1995) The effect of a child's hospitalisation on the parental role. *Professional Nurse*, 10(9), 561–3.

Foster, R., Hunsberger, M. and Anderson, J. (1989) *Family Centred Nursing Care for Children*, W.B. Saunders, Philadelphia.

Fradd, E. (1986) It's child's play. *Nursing Times*, 82(41), 40–42.

Fradd, E. (1996) The Importance of Negotiating a Care Plan. *Paediatric Nursing*, 8(6), 6–9.

Galvin, J. and Goldstone, L. (1988) *Junior Monitor*, Polytechnic Products Ltd, Newcastle upon Tyne.

Glen, S.A. (1982) Hospital admission through the parents' eyes. *Nursing Times*, 78(31), 1321–3.

Goodman, S. and Adams, C. (1989) 'Uncumphtable'. *Nursing Times*, 85(49), 28–31.

Hardgrove, C.B. and Dawson, R.B. (1972) *Parents and Children in the Hospital: The Family's Role in Pediatrics*, Little, Brown and Co, Boston.

Harris, P.J. (1979) *Children, their Parents and Hospital*, Unpublished PhD thesis, University of Nottingham.

Harris, P.J. (1981a) A link-person. *Nursing Times*, 77(44), 1891–2.

Harris, P.J. (1981b) Preparation of parents and their children for a planned hospital admission. *Nursing Times*, 77(41), 1744–6.

Harris, P.J. (1981c) Organisation of nursing duties and training. *Nursing Times*, 77(45), 1936–7.

Harvey, S. (1966) *Play in Hospital*, Heron, London.

Jolly, J. (1981) *The Other Side of Paediatrics*, Macmillan, London.

Jolly, J. (1988) Meeting the special needs of children in hospital. *Senior Nurse*, 8(4), 6–7.

Lavelle, J. (1994) Education and the sick child, in *Caring for dying children and their families*, (ed. L. Hill), Chapman and Hall, London.

McQuaid, L. (1996) Professional Role of the Children's Nurse, in *Children's Nursing*, (eds L. McQuaid, S. Husband and E. Parker), Churchill Livingstone, Edinburgh.

Morrison, L. (1997) Stress and Siblings. *Paediatric Nursing*, 9(4), 26–7.

Moss, J.R. (1981) Helping young children to cope with the physical examination. *Pediatric Nursing*, 7(17–20).

National Association for the Welfare of Children in Hospital (1984a) *Update No. 12: Summer,* NAWCH, London.

National Association for the Welfare of Children in Hospital (1984b) *Update No. 11: Spring,* NAWCH, London.

National Association for the Welfare of Children in Hospital (1986) *Review. NAWCH Update, Autumn 1986*, NAWCH, London.

National Association for the Welfare of Children in Hospital (1988) *NAWCH Quality Checklist: Caring for Children in Hospital*, NAWCH, London.

National Association for the Welfare of Children in Hospital (1989) *NAWCH Quality Review*, NAWCH, London.

Perthen, C. (1990) Involving the parents. *Nursing*, Series 4(19), 12–16.

Poster, E.C. (1983) Stress immunization: techniques to help children cope with hospitalization. *Maternal–Child Nursing Journal*, **12**, 119–34.

Robbins, M. (1987) The role of the nurse. *Nursing Series*, 3(24), 905–7.

Robinson, S. and Collier, J. (1997) Holding Children Still for Procedures. *Paediatric Nursing*, 9(4), 12–4.

Rodin, J. (1983) *Will This Hurt?* RCN, London.

Royal College of Nursing (1990) *Standards of Care: Paediatric Nursing*, RCN, London.

Rutter, M. (1981) *Maternal Deprivation Reassessed*, 2nd edn, Penguin, Harmondsworth.

Sadler, S. (1988) Being there. *Nursing Times*, 84(34), 19.

Smith, F. (1997) Children's Rights in Accident and Emergency Services. *Paediatric Nursing*, 9(9), 22–4.

Swanwick, M.M. (1996) Child-Rearing Across Cultures. *Paediatric Nursing*, 8(7), 13–15.

Weller, B. (1980) *Helping Sick Children Play*, Baillière Tindall, London.

Williams, J. (1989) Junior monitor: measuring standards of child care. *Nursing Times*, 85(29), 52.

Williamson, H. and Williamson, P. (1987) Coping with a child in hospital: the parents' view. *Nursing*, Series 3(24), 902–4.

Woodfield, T. (1997) Parents of Critically Ill Children: Do we meet their needs? *Paediatric Nursing*, 9(8), 22–4.

Consumers' Association (1980 and 1985) *Children in Hospital* (Consumer Reports), Consumers' Association, London.

Many of the findings of these reports have been discussed in this chapter, but we could not do justice to the illustrative power of the quotes which make up much of the substance. Both reports are certainly worth a thorough reading.

National Association for the Welfare of Children in Hospital now renamed *Action for Sick Children*, Argyle House, 300 Kingston Road, Wimbledon Chase, London SW20 8LX.

This association produces a range of excellent leaflets and reading lists on all aspects of the care of children in hospital.

Taylor, J. and Müller, D. (1995) *Nursing Adolescents: Research and Psychological Perspectives*, Blackwell, Oxford.

It has not been possible to give full consideration in this chapter to the adolescent although we do expand in chapter 10. This text however really does do justice to the care of the adolescent both in hospital and the community.

Warnock, H.N. (1978) *Special Educational Needs: Report of the Committee of Enquiry into the Education of Handicapped Children and Young People*, HMSO, London.

10 The Adolescent in Hospital

The major problem to be faced in trying to understand the needs of adolescents in hospital is that very little research has been carried out in this field. Much of the research which has been carried out is reviewed by Taylor and Müller (1995). There are theories about adolescent development (Coleman and Hendry, 1990), but they have not always been subjected to rigorous testing. There are also articles based on nurses' experiences of nursing adolescents which can be helpful, but these do not always have an objective basis. There is clearly room for nurses to carry out research with this important group of health care subscribers particularly as they are gradually receiving greater recognition within the health services as an homogenous group with very specific needs. Systematic investigation is required to give providers evidence which can inform both change and practice.

Growing and changing

Adolescence is often described as a 'passing phase' by weary parents, concerned teachers and health professionals; an interlude or transition between two important periods of life, childhood and adulthood. This can imply that it has no value of its own, and that it is just a period of waiting. This seems to be reflected in our tradition in hospitals, of treating adolescents in either children's or adults' wards. There are a growing number of adolescent wards in general hospitals but these are still the exception rather than the norm, although some children's departments do make real attempts to provide for adolescents by segregating them from younger children by, for example, allocating separate bays and bathrooms. Adolescence, however, is a period lasting up to about 10 years, and it is therefore surprising that we rarely view it in hospitals as a distinctive period.

Our traditional approach to nursing adolescents means that all nurses in training are likely to come across adolescent patients. For example, many road accidents and sporting injuries affect this age group, sometimes resulting in months in hospital and outpatients follow-up. Surgery of various kinds (e.g. appendectomy) is needed by many adolescents and some individuals will have had chronic medical conditions such as asthma and diabetes as children. These patients will usually progress from children's to adult wards as they grow older (or larger). There is a small but significant number of attempted suicides among adolescents, necessitating admission to general and psychiatric hospitals, and Taylor and Müller (1995) found that problems of antisocial behaviour, anorexia nervosa, depressive conditions and emotional disorders peak during adolescence.

This marks out adolescence as a time when problems are apparently typical, as earlier writers such as Hall at the turn of the century also suggested. Taylor and Müller (1995), summarizing Hall's work, describe his view of adolescence as a time of conflict between biological and cultural forces. The term 'storm and stress' has often been used to characterize this view of adolescence. Such a view may exaggerate the nature of adolescence and because some people have problems in this age group, necessitating psychiatric help, much of the research into adolescent development has focused on clinical samples, that is those needing help. It is dangerous to generalize from this that problems are typical of adolescence, and there is a risk of stereotyping.

Another approach to understanding adolescent development comes from ethology which we described in Chapter 1 in relation to the survival value of infant behaviours. Weisfield and Berger (1983) studied human and primate adolescents to compare their behaviour and development. One important feature of human and primate adolescence concerns physical changes, including the growth spurt at puberty, especially in males. It is at this time that they need to develop rapidly in order to become independent, capable of protecting themselves and of reproducing. In growing suddenly they become big enough to do this and reduce the time in which they may be vulnerable. Although these processes are biological, there may be social influences. Weisfield and Berger (1983) report that when the most dominant male in a troop of monkeys was removed, another male gained weight dramatically and the pattern was repeated in other males as the most dominant was removed. Working from this set of evidence, Weisfield and Berger suggested that in humans the pubertal growth spurt is part of an abrupt increase in preparedness for independence and reproduction. They propose also that behaviour, anatomy and culture are interacting aspects of the same purposeful development and that it is linked with the wellbeing of the population.

Perhaps the most influential approach to understanding adolescence is Erikson's theoretical work on psychosocial development (see, for example, Erikson, 1965). Adolescence has become associated with the process of acquiring identity and it is described as a 'task' of adolescence; something that everyone does during this period of their lives. Marcia (1982) points out that, though it is distinctive of adolescence, it is not exclusive to it. As he says (p. 159):

if the termination of adolescence were to depend on ... the formation of an identity, then, for some, it would never end.

What then do we mean by adolescence? We have already seen that it is a time associated with psychological and physical changes, which usually occur between about 10 and 20 years of age. Physiologically it begins around puberty, with the onset of menstruation in females and the production of live sperm in males. However, for psychologists, adolescence is not so much an age range in which physiological changes take place, but rather a developmental process. During this period psychological changes take place so that adult behaviours take over from the more childish ones. It is a 'process' rather than a 'stage' because there are a variety of adjustments to be made which may take months or years in each individual. There is no clearcut ending to adolescence, although the law reflects society's perceptions of adult status; we may marry at 16 years of age, hold a driving licence at 17 years and vote at 18 years of age. Social activities including marriage, house ownership and having children, are undertaken by different people at very different times. The specific beginning and ending of adolescence are perhaps rather less important than the characteristics within it and this is the subject matter for the remainder of this chapter.

THE PROCESS OF ADOLESCENCE

It would appear from the literature about adolescence that adults are people who have to some degree gained a sense of their own identity, while adolescents are more in the process of doing so. Marcia (1982) observes that the better developed one's sense of identity is the more aware one is both of one's own uniqueness and one's similarity to others, as well as of personal strengths and weaknesses. On the other hand, the less well developed this sense of identity is, the more confused individuals seem to be about their own distinctiveness from others and the more they rely on outside sources to evaluate themselves. However, identity is not something one possesses like red hair or a temper. It is a dynamic process which begins when the infant first recognizes its separateness from the primary caregiver and progresses by means of phases of development. Adolescence seems to be a crucial phase in which changes occur in relation to identity.

Marcia (1982) describes identity as 'an internal, self-constructed, dynamic organization of drives, abilities, beliefs and individual history'. The study of adolescence reveals those areas in which the construction of identity is concerned: values, politics, ethics, morals, thought processes, sexuality, friendship, intimate relationships. Although adolescence is primarily associated with identity changes, these may also continue to old age. The importance of identity in adolescence, according to Marcia, is that this is the first time that physical development, cognitive skills and social expectations coincide to enable young persons to understand their past and begin to decide upon their approach to the future. Often the process of developing identity is not conscious and decisions are rarely taken irrevocably. Instead, in response to experiences, decisions are made, then remade as necessary. It is in this sense that identity and adolescence are processes. They involve being open to change, developing toward goals, modifying ideas, establishing priorities and trying out various attitudes towards life. Marcia (1982) discusses these issues in detail and readers wishing to study this area further are encouraged to refer to this source.

An aim of nursing, already referred to in this book, is the maintenance of optimal physiological, psychological and spiritual functioning of patients. This implies that nurses need more knowledge of adolescent behaviour and development, rather than the occasional experience of nursing a teenager in an adult, paediatric, or obstetric ward. But what constitutes optimal physiological and psychological functioning in adolescence? The literature typically refers to a series of 'developmental tasks' (see, for example, McKinney *et al.*, 1977; Rogers, 1981; Taylor and Müller, 1995). The following discussion is based on McKinney *et al.* and may help in identifying some main aspects of development in adolescence, although it should not be regarded as exhaustive.

DEVELOPMENTAL TASKS FOR ADOLESCENTS

There appear to be a number of developmental tasks for adolescents including:

1. adjusting to a rapidly changing physique and sexual development;
2. achieving a sense of independence from parents;
3. acquiring the social skills of a young adult.
4. developing the necessary academic and vocational skills;
5. achieving a sense of oneself as a worthwhile person; and
6. achieving an internalized set of guiding norms and values.

Seen as a list like this it may appear that the process of adolescence is quite straightforward, but adolescents are not given such a list and told to work through it for 10 years! The list is simply a description of what many adolescents seem to do, and it may provide a useful basis for examining the possible effects of illness or hospitalization during adolescence. It is important to remember that there is a lack of research in this area and so many of the points made here are based on people's experiences of nursing adolescents, and have not always been tested empirically.

Adjusting to a rapidly changing physique and to sexual development

Alsaker (1996), when discussing the impact of puberty, suggests that it is not just the changes themselves which are important but the context of the changes which will influence adjustment. Alsaker discusses differences between adolescents including how they perceive puberty, how they interpret the physical changes, and what expectations they have.

Commonsense suggests that this aspect of adolescence affects various features of hospitalization. Physical examinations, treatments and maintaining hygiene can all provoke embarrassment for the adolescent who may not have adjusted fully to bodily changes. Mitchell (1980) showed that younger male adolescents were much more concerned about touch at medical examination than older adolescents who had already come to terms with their new physique and bodily sensations.

She pointed out, though, that many female health professionals use touch as a form of communication, especially to reassure, and that this could be disturbing for young male adolescents. In this research the subjects were healthy and it might be different if the subjects were ill or suffering. Mitchell also emphasized the importance of using appropriate encounters with adolescents to help stimulate and develop their interest in the functioning of the body, with the view to promoting a healthy approach to living. This is a consistent theme found in the literature and assumptions are frequently made that adolescents are negligent of health, but interested in themselves. Miles and Eid (1997) found that, in relation to healthy eating, this was indeed the case, although the negligence was not through lack of knowledge but rather that adolescents saw the problem as 'belonging too far in the future to relate it to their lives now' (p. 48). They suggest that practitioners should use educational opportunities to convince adolescents of the relevance of healthy eating to themselves. Leyn (1980) suggests 'appealing to adolescents' natural developmental narcissism' (pp. 32–33) to draw them into an alliance with the nurse to preserve physical and emotional wellbeing and to educate them concerning care for their bodies. Again this implies that problems are anticipated but preventable, though it may be based on assumptions and stereotypes rather than on a real appraisal of the development of healthy adolescents.

Another theme emerging from the literature suggests that adolescents are normally preoccupied with adjusting to their developing bodies and new sensations. One writer, Savedra (1979), believed that when illness or an accident caused them to experience new sensations such as pain and discomfort, they became confused by what is an effect of illness and what is a normal sensation. This she suggested may lead to reactions being out of proportion to the actual biological condition. On the other hand, it is increasingly clear that at any age experience affects reactions to suffering and pain and that people express suffering according to their cultural background (McCavery, 1985). It is rather bold to state therefore that adolescent reactions are merely part of an adjustment to their changing physique and emerging sexuality. A further suggestion by Savedra (1979) was that adolescence is a time associated with a rich fantasy life, which in some instances enables the adolescent to imagine dire consequences out of proportion to the illness or injury. On the other hand, adolescents may deny the severity of their ill health (see Cowen *et al.*, 1986; MacKenzie, 1988; Taylor and Müller, 1995). Helping adolescents through denial is an important goal of nursing care and it may be necessary to seek skilled help for the adolescent whilst they are in this phase. Denial of ill health may or may not be more true of adolescents than the rest of the population. Without research evidence it is difficult to be sure. It would, at a commonsense level, underline the importance of giving clear and straightforward information to adolescents who are ill, allowing plenty of scope for discussion and providing well designed information which they can follow up at their leisure.

A concern with appearance is an important part of physical development, though the somewhat stereotyped idea of adolescents as permanently peering into mirrors may have exaggerated its significance. Nurses writing about adolescence seem to describe acute self-consciousness as typical and encourage other nurses to remember to knock before entering bathrooms, and to understand how difficult it is for this age group to cope with bed pans and commodes. They suggest 'engaged' signs for doors which cannot be locked. However, such measures seem to be appropriate for all patients not just for adolescents. Perhaps this emphasis arises from treating adolescents in open children's wards where there is a particular shortage of private, personal space and where patients have limited control over their environment. It is reasonable to state that illness or injury which affects appearance or sexuality will require particular understanding from caregivers. A common theme in the literature concerns the significance to adolescents of both sexes of even a single facial spot. The assumption therefore is that a disfiguring injury will be almost impossible to cope with. This may be the case, but it may be too simple a view. The actual reactions of individuals will depend on a number of factors such as whether their condition is chronic or acute, of recent onset or long term, what sort of support family and friends can give and the personality and attitudes of the person affected. We should probably not take too narrow a view of the individual consequences of disfigurement for adolescents. While seeking deep appreciation of the personal meanings of an illness or injury for a particular adolescent, we should probably not assume or imply that adolescents are ill equipped to cope with disruption of the developmental task of adjusting to bodily changes and sexuality.

Achieving independence from parents

In early adolescence, new styles of friendship develop. A really close friend with whom to share a deepest secret thought becomes very important, according to Fine (1980). His research into boys' friendships indicates that groups spend quite a lot of time in aggressive and sexual 'naughty talk' which they would not engage in with parents. Young adolescents seem to need same-sex company and may perhaps find mixed wards very difficult to cope with, though older adolescents may prefer this since their friendship patterns typically include members of both sexes.

Being in hospital may affect adolescents' dependence on their parents in different ways (MacKenzie, 1988). For some it may make them feel more dependent, particularly if it is necessary for parents to start or continue physical care. For others the enforced separation may actually help some adolescents to gain independence and it is clearly both difficult and undesirable to make generalizations. This brings us back to one of our dominant themes throughout this book which is the importance of individualized care and assessment. Nurses should not make assumptions about a particular relationship an adolescent has with his or her parents or indeed that an adolescent will react in a particular way in a particular set of circumstances. Howe *et al.* (1993), for example, found that there were several factors which might influence the adolescent. These factors include the particular domain of functioning being studied as well as gender and age and whether the adolescent has a neurological disorder. For example, boys with neurological disorders experienced greater problems than girls. Howe *et al.* (1993, p. 1167) write:

> *Adolescent development is multifaceted: general factors such as family burden may have important effects on some facets of development, factors specific to the general category of condition (such as brain based conditions) may have important effects in still other facets, and factors specific to particular disease entities may have unique effects in still other domains.*

A typical view of parent–adolescent relations is one of conflict. However, Anderson and Clarke (1982) describe studies concluding that conflict is not typical. Increasingly, though, where it does occur it may be different for males compared with females. They cite one study which showed that conflict with boys concerned independence of action and freedom of movement, while for girls it was concerned with their desire to be themselves and not feel threatened by the influence and forcefulness of their parents. An important way of promoting independence is through involving adolescent patients in discussions and decisions about their care and treatment (Gillies, 1992). Some adolescents will continue to involve parents, others may not, and it may be the case that some will vary from day to day. Caregivers then will need to develop great sensitivity towards each individual and try to build up trust. The literature concerned with nursing adolescents encourages nurses to adopt an open, frank and sensitive approach to their questions (spoken and unspoken). If adolescents experience difficulty in knowing how to achieve independence from parents, parents too seem to experience difficulty in knowing how to help them. This can put nurses in a difficult position and calls for very good communication between all parties.

Acquiring the social skills of a young adult

Social skills develop through contact with other people, but certain groups of people are socially isolated from time to time. The elderly, the chronically ill and the disabled may be among these, perhaps because of reduced mobility. There is a risk for anyone hospitalized for a long time, that visitors may cease to call, or conversations become difficult because the patient may feel they have little if any news, and little relevant contact with the world outside. Some people may need little social contact and yet be satisfied, whilst others may receive quite a lot, but still feel lonely. The kind of social interaction people need seems to vary with age. Anderson and Clarke (1982) suggest that adolescents preferred contact with other young people, while elderly people preferred contact with their families. They cite studies of how normal adolescents spend their leisure time. Contact with peers outside school hours was very high, while only a few went out regularly with parents. Many belonged to clubs, spent time reading, watching television and going to see films.

In contrast, disabled adolescents in Anderson and Clarke's (1982) study had very limited social lives. Many rarely saw friends outside school, especially if they themselves attended special schools. Others went out regularly with parents, especially those attending special schools. Here too they watched far more television, but spent less time reading or engaged in hobbies. They did belong to clubs in the special schools, but these were often solely for the disabled and only during term time. In this study, parents and teachers thought that the disabled adolescents had difficulties with peer relationships more often than did non-disabled adolescents. They were described as solitary, preferring to be alone. When asked what difficulties their disabled offspring had, parents usually mentioned shyness, lack of self-confidence and self-consciousness. These are problems which are thought to affect many normal adolescents, not just those who have physical problems. Therefore, if in the disabled such difficulties are preventing social inter-action and leading to solitary behaviour, it may be that these adolescents are being hindered in developing the social skills of young adults.

It is difficult to generalize about the best ways to help adolescents in hospital because, again, circumstances will affect each patient differently. One principle, which seems sensible, is to try and relate to adolescents as people to be taken seriously. A practical example might be to take their history on admission not only with the parent, but also from the adolescent alone. Dragone (1990) in her study of chronically ill adolescents and their parents found variations in their perspectives about the difficulties and needs of the adolescent. It is important for the nurse to be aware of both perspectives. In addition, it is possible that adolescents will regard some of their experiences as personal and confidential and not to be discussed with parents. Granting them, where possible, the confidentiality expected by adults may help them to develop maturity in dealing with matters concerning their own health and illness, and thus help them acquire adult social skills. It is important, however, that nurses are aware of relevant legislation when caring for adolescents and important changes were introduced by the Children Act of 1989. Issues relating to legal aspects of nursing care are fully discussed by Dimond (1996).

Developing the necessary academic and vocational skills

Choosing employment and developing academic and vocational skills are important features of adolescence. It can be acutely distressing if hospitalization disrupts plans and examinations, and it is helpful to try and ascertain the effect of hospitalization on individuals' lives at the time in order to understand and support them. The adolescent (as described in Chapter 4) becomes capable of thinking in abstract, or hypothetical terms, and can now imagine 'as if' situations relating to illness and injury which are not actually part of their experience of life so far. Thus, adolescents with a disability may re-interpret what have become common place experiences (Birchenall, 1995) and start to view them in the light of future relationships and work prospects.

In hospital, it should be possible to give adolescents' educational requirements priority in care planning. Orthopaedic patients, for example, are often well but immobile, and careful planning with support from hospital teachers and the patient's school should enable studying to continue with minimal disruption. Thompson (1990) in her discussion about the needs of children with cancer emphasizes the importance of continued schooling for adolescents and Fradd (1986) finds that teachers can provide a semblance of normality in an otherwise disordered world. However, in a Save the Children Fund Survey (1989) it was found that there are considerable variations in the number and qualifications of teachers working in hospitals. Over 44 per cent had a background in infant teaching which may mean they have limited experience of adolescent needs. Teachers from the patient's own school are often keen to help and Thompson (1990) suggests that if teachers do make contact with the hospital it is a good opportunity for nurses to answer questions within the bounds of confidentiality and prepare for the return of the adolescent to school following discharge. Ensuring teachers are aware of facts, rather than hearsay should help the adolescent and prevent the teacher adopting an overprotective attitude which Thompson warns can lead to the adolescent adopting the 'sick role'.

Hospitalization may be inevitable and may disrupt an individual's plans, but such plans are still an important part of life for the adolescent in hospital. Whether or not they are maintained, modified or abandoned may depend to some extent on the interest caregivers have in the individual's future beyond a spell in hospital. Since adolescence is a time in which it seems to be important to make plans and work towards some future occupational goal, nurses may be able to enhance the process by their recognition that it needs to take place, their understanding of its difficulties and their willingness to try and support their adolescent patients. Blunden (1989) writes that adolescents should be:
... invited to give information about their lives at home and school, about their goals, concerns, knowledge of their illness and expectations of health care.

Achieving a sense of oneself as a worthwhile person

Many adolescents hold very strong views concerning political or religious issues and, if they see things in rather black and white terms, may be perturbed by the conflicts they encounter within and around themselves. Many try at this time to contribute to solving community problems, others work voluntarily in homes for disabled and elderly people. These kinds of activities can give a sense of being a worthwhile person, but for the adolescent who has a chronic illness or disability there may be an overwhelming sense of being a burden and great difficulty in ever finding the opportunity to develop a sense of self worth through such activities. It would seem to be important for nurses admitting such patients to their wards to have in mind this need for self worth and to consider the nature of their own worth in relation to being the giver of care. It may be especially important to encourage the adolescent patient to take an active rather than passive role in care (Gillies, 1992). For example, as noted earlier, self worth may be enhanced by involving adolescents in discussions and decisions about how their particular care will be planned and carried out.

Achieving an internalized set of guiding norms and values

This refers to being able to make one's own decisions about all sorts of issues and is part of the socialization process of acquiring attitudes and values which are compatible with those of society. For many, adolescence is a time for experimenting and testing family or community norms and values. Rapoport and Rapoport (1980) put it this way (p. 97):

> *The ultimate aim of any process of socialization should be to permit each adolescent to develop his or her unique potential as a human being, consistent with the rights of others.*

A period of hospitalization could enhance or disrupt this process, depending on whether the environment is designed to allow such processes to continue. Hospitals typically impose norms and values on the people they care for, but perhaps those staff caring for adolescents need to think through the implications of such traditions for adolescent development.

MAINTAINING THE PROCESS OF ADOLESCENCE

In discussing various developmental tasks in adolescence, it is obvious that there is overlap. This indicates the difficulty of trying to break down the process of adolescence for discussion, and highlights the integrated nature of the developmental process. However, developmental tasks do serve as a rough guide to some of the issues faced by adolescents, and to the implications of aiming to maintain optimal psychological functioning in individuals. Many writers suggest that providing separate adolescent units is the answer to maintaining the process of adolescence in hospital. However, in Blunden's study (1989), which looked at where adolescents would *prefer* to be nursed, she found that children's preferences changed dramatically between the ages of 11 and 13 years, with 80.8 per cent of 11 year olds preferring to be nursed on a children's ward and 100 per cent of over 13 year olds preferring an adolescent ward. While it may be advantageous to offer specialized units and staff (and there are a growing number of designated units nationally), it should not be regarded as impossible to maintain optimal psychological functioning in adolescents where special provision is impossible. It does seem that well prepared staff with appropriate skills and knowledge about adolescence could provide good care whatever the architectural arrangements in the hospital. What is required is a degree of self motivation among all staff to read and develop an understanding of the process of adolescence, and to try and bring this to their patients in whatever setting. There are also a number of post registration programmes which look specifically at aspects of working with adolescents.

One final point of discussion which is perhaps of equal importance to the transition from childhood to adolescence is the issue of transferring adolescents with chronic illnesses from children's health care services to adult services which are differently structured and most probably more impersonal. One interesting project in South England focussed on this theme with the aim of providing guidelines for good practice, setting clear evidence based targets and auditable outcomes. The contributions to the project are brought together in a collection of papers edited by Kurtz and Hopkins (1996). It is essential reading for any health care practitioner involved in any way with adolescent users of the health services.

We have considered the developmental tasks of adolescence which, taking place at and around a period of immense physical change, constitute the psychological process of development from childhood to adulthood. Hopefully we have demonstrated some of the implications for nurses of aiming to maintain optimal physiological and psychological functioning in adolescent patients. Some practical implications are set out below, but it is emphasized that this chapter can only serve as an introduction to a very important and neglected area in health care. Research too in the area is somewhat limited. Adolescents may seem to be the 'Cinderellas' of the National Health Service, but nurses have a marvellous opportunity to develop expertise in this field, and initiate research to help in the quest for better care. We offer some useful sources for further reading and hope that these will encourage and stimulate a lively interest in adolescents in the minds of many nurses. Finally, it should be said that almost all nurses in training are themselves adolescents, and it would perhaps help them to become more aware of the process through which they have recently been progressing. Whether or not nurses are developmentally ready to try and nurse patients who are also adolescents is beyond the scope of this chapter, but it may be useful to give some thought to this matter.

In practice ➤

- Nurses should try to create an appropriate environment to allow adolescent development to progress. This should offer privacy, somewhere for peer interaction, appropriate materials such as radios, computers, mirrors, cosmetics, magazines, puzzles, and games for groups (e.g. a pool table). A kitchen and opportunities to make drinks and snacks are also recommended.
- Information relevant to the priorities of adolescence should be offered. For example, fact sheets concerning aspects of health care and sexual development. The effects and meanings of

conditions and treatments (especially if visible) should be anticipated and adolescents helped to understand the normal functions of their bodies, and the changes introduced by puberty, or a medical condition.

- Independence should be promoted by establishing trust and encouraging the adolescent to take responsibility in decision making regarding aspects of nursing care and treatment. Ways of assisting adolescents to develop their own set of rules and attitudes without compromising others should be found. For example establishing rules for lights out and morning waking.
- Nurses should consider how the hospitalized adolescent can, despite a degree of dependency, still feel worthwhile as a person. The typical active role of the nurse and passive role of the patient, particularly in the case of long term patients, should be reassessed. For example, could the roles be developed or modified to enable individual adolescents to offer help to others? What are their gifts regardless of their illness or disability? Can these be enhanced?
- Nurses need to understand the possible reactions of adolescents to hospitalization, for example, regressing to more childlike behaviours, and thus reverting to earlier forms of dependence on parents, vacillating between adult and childlike behaviours, denying the extent of an illness and others.
- The social needs of adolescents need accommodating by for example encouraging private visits from close friends and perhaps small groups of peers from school.
- Disruption of school courses and examinations should be prevented by providing access to teaching staff and facilities for study if the patient can manage to do some. Goals and aspirations should be discussed especially where these may be affected by hospitalization or the patient's condition.

REFERENCES

Alsaker, F.D. (1996) The Impact of Puberty. *Journal of Child Psychology and Psychiatry*, 37(3), 249–58.

Anderson, E.M. and Clarke, L. (1982) *Disability in Adolescence*, Methuen, London.

Birchenall, M. (1995) Disability: An Issue for the Growing Child, in *Childhood to Adolescence: Caring for Health*, (A. Fatchett), Baillière Tindall, London.

Blunden, R. (1989) An artificial state. *Paediatric Nursing*, 1(1), 12–13.

Coleman, J. and Hendry, L. (1990) *The nature of Adolescence*, Routledge, London.

Cowen, L., Mok, J., Corey, M., MacMillan, H., Simmons, R. and Levison, H. (1986) Psychologic adjustments of the family with a member who has cystic fibrosis. *Pediatrics*, 77(5), 745–53.

Dimond, B. (1996) *The Legal Aspects of Child Health Care*, Mosby, London.

Dragone, M.A. (1990) Perspectives of chronically ill adolescents and parents on health care needs. *Pediatric Nursing*, 16(1), 45–50.

Erikson, E. (1965) *Childhood and Society*, Penguin, Harmondsworth.

Fine, G.A. (1980) The natural history of preadolescent male friendship groups, in *Friendship and Social Relations in Children*, (eds H.C. Foot, A.J. Chapman and J.R. Smith), John Wiley, Chichester.

Fradd, E. (1986) It's child's play. *Nursing Times*, 82(41), 40–42.

Gillies, M. (1992) Teenage Trauma. *Nursing Times*, 88(27), 26–29.

Howe, G.W., Feinstein, C., Reiss, D., Molock, S. and Berger, K. (1993) Adolescent Adjustment to Chronic Physical Disorders – I: Comparing Neurological and Non Neurological Conditions. *Journal of Child Psychology and Psychiatry*, 34(7), 1153–71.

Kurtz, Z. and Hopkins, A. (eds) (1996) *Services for Young People with Chronic Disorders: in their transition from childhood to adult life*, Royal College of Physicians, London.

Leyn, R.B. (1980) The nurse–adolescent relationship, in *Nursing Care of Adolescents*, (J. Howe), McGraw-Hill, New York.

MacKenzie, H. (1988) Teenagers in hospital. *Nursing Times*, 84(32), 58–61.

Marcia, J.E. (1982) Identity in adolescence, in *Handbook of Adolescent Psychology*, (ed. J. Anderson), John Wiley, Chichester.

McCavery, R. (1985) Spiritual care in acute illness, in *Nursing and Spiritual Care*, (eds O. McGilloway and F. Myco), Harper & Row, London.

McKinney, J.P., Fitzgerald, H.E. and Strommen, E.A. (1977) *The Adolescent and Young Adult*, Dorsey Press, Illinois.

Miles, G. and Eid, S. (1997) The Dietary Habits of Young People. *Nursing Times*, 93(50), 46–8.

Mitchell, J.R. (1980) Male adolescents' concern about a physical examination conducted by a female. *Nursing Research*, 29, 165–9.

Rapoport, R. and Rapoport, R. (1980) *Growing Through Life*, Harper & Row, London.

Rogers, D. (1981) *Adolescents and Youth*, Prentice Hall, Englewood Cliffs, NJ.

Savedra, M. (1979) The adolescent in hospital, in *Perspectives in Adolescent Health Care*, (ed. R.T. Mercer), J.B. Lippincott, Philadelphia.

Save the Children Fund (1989) Play provision in hospital. *Paediatric Nursing*, 1(3), 19–20.

Taylor, J. and Müller, D. (1995) *Nursing Adolescents: Research and Psychological Perspectives*, (ed. J. Thompson), Blackwell, Oxford.

Thompson, J. (1990) The adolescent with cancer, in *The Child with Cancer*, (ed. J. Thompson), Scutari Press, London.

Weisfield, E. and Berger, J.M. (1983) Some features of human adolescence viewed in evolutionary perspective. *Human Development*, 26, 121–33.

FURTHER READING

Anderson, E.M. and Clarke, L. (1982) *Disability in Adolescence*, Methuen, London.

A very useful research study comparing disabled and non-disabled subjects regarding developmental tasks.

Kurtz, Z. and Hopkins, A. (eds) (1996) *Services for Young People with Chronic Disorders: in their transition from childhood to adult life*, Royal College of Physicians, London.

An excellent collection of papers relating to the difficulties of adolescents as they move towards adulthood and adult focussed health services.

Taylor, J. and Müller, D. (1995) *Nursing Adolescents: Research and Psychological Perspectives*, Blackwell, Oxford.

A comprehensive text covering a spectrum of issues relating to adolescents in health and illness including developmental aspects.

Vaughan, V.C. and Litt, I.F. (1990) *Child and Adolescent Development: Clinical Implications*, T.B. Saunders, Philadelphia.

A comprehensive book about physical and psychological aspects of adolescence. An excellent source book for health carers involved with adolescents.

NURSING ILL CHILDREN IN THE COMMUNITY

In Part Two so far we have focussed on the child in hospital and how hospitalization can affect both the child's development and his or her relationships with siblings and parents. There are, however, many ill children and adolescents who can be cared for successfully without needing to spend excessive time in hospital. These include:

1. children with acute ill health or short term health problems;
2. children with chronic ill health or longer term health problems; and
3. dying children who wish to spend their remaining life at home.

The aim of this chapter is to look at the psychological needs of ill children and their families in the community. Empirical data about the benefits of home care as compared to hospital care are, however, limited and only a few small-scale evaluative studies have been undertaken in this field. There remains a need for larger scale comparative studies, which look at issues such as quality of care, child and family satisfaction and the psychological and social implications of community care for the family.

ALTERNATIVES TO HOSPITAL CARE

In Chapter 7 the adverse effects of hospitalization have been fully discussed. The Platt report (1959) recognized the psychological trauma of children spending time in hospital and recommended the setting up of a specialist nursing service for the home care of children. This report was published in the era of Bowlby's (1951) influential work on the detrimental effects of separation of young children from their mothers and Robertson's work (see Robertson and Robertson, 1989) about the effects of institution care. Very few health districts followed the recommendations of the Platt report and set up home care schemes and in 1976 the Court report reiterated the need to look at the community care of sick children, as did the Department of Health (1991) and the Audit Commission (1993).

The situation remained somewhat disappointing. Whiting's (1989) study, which looked at community nursing provision for children nationally, showed that by 1988 only 12.6 per cent (n = 23) of district health authorities had a community child care nursing team. Another 17.4 per cent of districts had plans to introduce teams. The teams that were in existence varied considerably in terms of the number of qualified children's nurses, with 11 'teams' consisting of a single nurse. The number of children seen and the type of referrals accepted also varied. The 'teams' which consisted of a single nurse were unable to provide 24 hour cover, in fact only one larger team was able to provide fully comprehensive cover. Where complete cover was not available, interim care was generally provided by generic district nursing colleagues. Tatman and Woodroffe in a second study in 1993 found that, whilst the situation had improved, the majority of areas in the country (70%) still had no comprehensive service. By 1996, whilst this figure had improved, 50 per cent of areas still had no service (Department of Health 1996).

It is not the intention to question the competence of interim care by non-children's trained nurses, but if community children's nursing care is to be advanced as a true alternative to hospital care then the children must be afforded the same rights as children who receive care in hospital. Action for Sick Children's charter, which was launched in 1984 under the NAWCH title, states that:

> *Children shall enjoy the care of appropriately trained staff, fully aware of the physical and emotional needs of each age group.*

This means nurses who are skilled in both community and child care nursing because, while paediatric nurses argue that children have special needs which require special skills, district nurses and health visitors equally may argue that nursing in the community also requires special skills. Indeed the Department of Health (1996) emphasizes this point by stating that community children's services should be 'led and predominantly staffed by nurses who possess both registration as a children's nurse and experience of community nursing'. The majority of RSCNs learned to nurse sick children in institutions and, although nurses trained under the Project 2000 scheme (UKCC, 1986) gain experience in both institutional and non-institutional settings, there is an urgent need to look at the educational requirements of already qualified paediatric nurses who wish to work within the community. One of the difficulties has been a lack of suitable training for such a role. However, what has emerged with the introduction of Community Specialist Practice (UKCC, 1994) is a defined programme of education which will qualify practitioners for community children's nursing and which will play 'a key role in shaping the health care of children as we move into the next millennium' (Langlands and McDonagh, 1995). However, what is apparent currently is that the shortage of appropriately qualified nurses is restraining the development of a nationwide service (*Paediatric Nursing* News, 1995).

IMPLICATIONS OF COMMUNITY CARE FOR THE CHILD AND FAMILY

Clearly, community nursing teams for ill children and adolescents will benefit many families who will not have to face excessive periods of time apart or face frequent visits to hospital for procedures that can be carried out successfully at home by suitably qualified nurses. More

children are able to have day surgery and others can be discharged home
earlier following major surgery. Children with acute and chronic medical
problems, premature babies who require long term care and dying
children can all spend less time in hospital. However, it must not be
assumed that community care is a feasible option for all families and we
should be aware of the implications of home care for the child, the
parents and the siblings.

Effects of home care on the child

The Action for Sick Children charter (1984) states:

> ...*children shall be admitted to hospital only if the care they require
> cannot equally well be provided at home or on a day basis.*

The benefits of home care for the child and adolescent are many.
Children who are able to have surgery on a day basis do not suffer from
excessive periods of separation from their families and should not be
subjected to some of the aspects of hospitalization to which we refer in
Chapter 7. Children can recover within the comfort of their own homes
in an environment where they feel secure.

Chapter 2 looks at the needs of newborn babies in relation to
attachment with their carers, and their perception of people and the
environment. The long term psychological effects of spending excessive
periods of time in neonatal units are not yet known and indeed most
pre-term babies are able to be discharged quite quickly (usually by the
time they reach term). Those who remain in neonatal units longer than
this often become labelled as 'geriatric neonates' (Sleath, 1994). Tew
(1994) suggests that these sick, very low birthweight babies may
experience severe problems on discharge. Community support can
enable these babies to be discharged home much earlier, with parents
and community child care nurses sharing the care. This will include an
increasing number of oxygen dependent babies who are discharged on
continuous oxygen therapy, often with skilled neonatal nurses providing
outreach services (Sleath, 1994). An earlier study in Canada by Lefebvre
and Bard (1983) showed that babies suffered no ill effects from being
discharged early and it was anticipated that the benefits would include
'favourable effects on long term parental–infant interaction'.
Community support can also enable parents to bring their dying babies
home so that they can spend their short lives with their families. A study
by Delight and Goodall (1988) which looked at palliative care of babies
with inoperable spina bifida emphasized the benefits of home care for
these babies and their parents.

> *It does help their self-esteem to know that having produced a child
> with a handicap they have nursed their child to the end.*

Children who have chronic ill health, such as cystic fibrosis or cancer,
can also benefit from community care particularly where generalist
nursing teams have support from nurse specialists who are generally

based in regional or sub-regional centres (Kelly *et al.*, 1994/5). Such relationships do exist particularly in relation to children's cancer services (Gould, 1996). The benefits of home care for children include the ability to be able regularly to attend schools and playgroups. Strehlow (1987) emphasizes that the school nurse can assist with children who have special needs, enabling them to continue at school while receiving relevant treatment and therapies during school time. This involves close liaison between the child, the parents, the school nurse and the community child care nurse. Parmelee (1989) suggests that if the parents of younger children with chronic illness or disabilities are not supported, their anxiety may result in the children finding it difficult to develop a strong 'sense of self'. This can affect their relationship with their parents and can also influence their behaviour when they experience subsequent health problems.

Maintaining children with chronic ill health at home, early discharge following surgery and day surgery do however have potential disadvantages. It can be very traumatic for the child to be discharged home unless it is quite clear what care is needed and what should be done if unexpected problems occur. If parents are anxious and do not feel confident in their abilities, children may become fearful. Glasper *et al.* (1989) emphasized the importance of being selective about which children are suitable candidates for early discharge or day surgery. Marland (1994) stressed that parents must be 'agreeable and prepared to accept responsibility for caring for the child within the home environment'. Relevant community resources must be readily available to the family. For example, Atwell and Gow (1985) emphasize that children and families will only benefit from day care if an 'efficient service' for caring for children at home is operational. Kitson *et al.* (1987) also identified that the quality of care could be affected if ward staff do not communicate with community staff and mobilize appropriate resources. However, Whiting's (1989) research shows that in many district health authorities there are no appropriately trained nurses employed within the community with whom hospital nurses can communicate. Clearly, until the number of community child care nursing teams increases and they are able to offer continuous cover, there will inevitably be children who have to spend excessive periods of time in hospital. Where teams do exist it is also vital that liaison between the various community disciplines is maintained e.g. between children's nurses and health visitors (Marland, 1994). Careful discharge planning is one area which is key to this (Bishop *et al*, 1994).

THE EFFECTS OF HOME CARE ON PARENTS AND SIBLINGS

Parmelee (1989) discusses the problems faced by parents and their ill children and emphasizes how difficult it is for them to retain confidence in themselves and each other when illness occurs. There is always the potential that, if illness in childhood is not 'handled' well, relationship disturbances will occur. Parmelee discusses minor illness which most children will suffer throughout their early years. The behaviour of parents to these transient minor episodes can greatly influence the child's ability to cope with more severe health problems. These findings have implications for community children's nurses and other community nurses. Health visitors, for example, are in the unique position of having access to families in 'health' and during minor illness. They have the opportunity to get to know families and gain knowledge of family dynamics. They should therefore be able to identify when family relationships are suffering after a child has been in hospital. Parents will need help to gain back their confidence after a child has been ill, especially if they have guilt feelings about the cause of the admission. Parmelee writes (1989, p. 151):

> *Those who advise parents must consciously help them work towards regaining confidence in their competence as caregivers and in their child's physical sturdiness.*

If health visitors have knowledge of existing family problems then it is important that visiting community child care nurses are made aware of difficulties. If relationship disturbances are present it could affect the way in which the child and the family react to the child's illness. Communication between visiting professionals must be effective. Parmelee reports that if episodes of ill health are managed well at home then it can give parents a strong sense of 'accomplishment' and will therefore strengthen the child–parent relationship. The child and the family can positively benefit from episodes of ill health.

Parents who care for dying children at home will also need the support of community nurses. Nurses can support parents, who may be involved in administering medication and providing other physical care. They can help parents through the emotional experience of answering the questions of both the ill child and any siblings. There is evidence to suggest that parents make better adaptations if they can care for their dying child at home. Lauer *et al.* (1983), in their studies of parental adaptation following the death of a child at home when compared to parents whose child had died in hospital, found that the home care parents experienced fewer feelings of guilt and fewer pathological grief reactions than the hospital group.

Sidey (1990), a community child care nurse, states that families should have the choice about whether they wish to care for a dying child at home. Not all parents will feel able to take on the responsibility. Sidey emphasizes that, at times in her experience, families have had to be denied home care in the interest of the child, where complex social problems exist. The physical needs of the child sometimes have to take precedence. Sidey also discusses the complex psychological needs of the dying child and the relationship of the child within the family. She describes (p. 11) one 7 year old child with cystic fibrosis who was denied the opportunity to discuss his own death:

> *He did go home and died 10 days later, afraid to lie down in case he*

died while asleep and asking me not to tell his mother he was dying. His chest was not as bad as some I have nursed, his nutrition was a problem and his morale rock bottom. His care was not a good example of cooperation, his death untimely and undignified. I hope we all learned a lot.

Without doubt, nurses involved with dying children and their families require many skills to care for their physical needs. However, they should also be able to recognize and care appropriately for psychological and social needs as well. The stress on the other members of the family involved with a dying child is great. Hicks (1989) discusses a family who had cared for a little girl who eventually died. The family separated after the death. Glasper *et al.* (1989) discuss the need to continue to visit bereaved families after the child's death for as long as the parents require the support.

Effects on siblings

As far as we know there is no work which looks directly at the effects on siblings of having an ill brother or sister who is being nursed at home as opposed to hospital, although many studies have looked at siblings' reactions to illness (see Chapter 3). Other studies have found evidence which relates to sibling behaviour which it is useful to look at here (Dunn, 1988; Dunn and Kendrick, 1982). Dunn and Kendrick (1982) looked at temperament in siblings when changes in the family occurred. They found, for example, that when a new baby was born, sibling inter-action with mothers altered and there were significant behavioural changes towards their mothers when mother and baby were interacting. Children who received the least attention from their mothers exhibited the most negative behaviour. There are studies which found similar problems in siblings when mothers had to spend time with ill children (Kohler and Radford, 1989). When the siblings were very young the problems appeared to be most acute (p. 322):

Young siblings are particularly vulnerable since they are most dependent on their mother. She (the mother) may be anxious to spend most of her time with the sick child, but frustrated by lack of time for the baby.

Kohler and Radford also discuss research which looks at the effect on siblings when a brother or sister dies. Allowing siblings to participate in care, giving them time to say 'goodbye' and allowing them to attend the funeral were found to help them adjust to the death, but the benefits to siblings if the brother or sister died at home as opposed to hospital were 'questionable'.

Bluebond-Langer (1989) also discusses the effects on siblings when a dying child is cared for at home. She describes siblings as living in 'houses of chronic sorrow', also mentioning the effects of reduced time and attention for their needs because of increased parental involvement with the dying child. Well siblings often experience changes in lifestyle, observe changes in their parents' emotions and cannot maintain normal friendship patterns with their peers. Bluebond-Langer suggests that they feel confused, rejected and lonely. However, McGowan (1994) found that siblings of children who died at home rather than in hospital adapted better.

So far in this section on siblings we have concentrated on the negative aspects of caring for sick children at home. Clearly there are also positive benefits for siblings if families remain at home rather than becoming fragmented when their ill brother or sister is hospitalized. This is especially true if a parent also stays in hospital, as time spent with the hospitalized child will further result in a lack of attention for the well siblings. Siblings may not only miss their parents but also their ill brother or sister. Cowen *et al*. (1986), in their study of the families of children with cystic fibrosis, found that pre-school siblings reacted negatively to the hospitalization of the ill child because of the temporary loss of their 'live in' playmate. Doyle (1987) suggests that siblings need help if they are to make successful adjustments to the experience of having an ill brother or sister. Community children's nurses and the health visitor should assess the family situation and account for the needs of siblings when planning care.

THE LOCUS OF CONTROL

Caring for an ill child at home requires motivation, skill and resources on the part of the parents. 'Partnership in care' is a popular phrase which has legal, ethical and psychological implications for the nurse, the child, the family and the employing health district. The partnership involves giving back control to parents or, in some instances, the child. Brykczynska (1987) sees partnerships with children as a way of treating the child as a developing individual who has rights within the partnership. One of these rights is that the nurse will not adopt a paternalistic role which affords a superior position and enables him or her to dictate care. The child is a co-worker, although parents maintain legal responsibility. In successful community care, multiple partnerships exist including those between specialist hospitals, District General Hospitals, community children's nurses, health visitors, parents, social service carers and other members of the primary health care team (Gould, 1996).

Partnerships with parents involve them taking back control for their ill child from nursing staff and this may seem an obvious move for them to want to make. However, for many parents who have to take on the responsibility for undertaking complicated technical care within the home, it is a move that requires great commitment. Nurses who work in acute hospital settings always have the option of handing back control, ultimately to the consultant, if they feel care is not within their competence (see Clause 4 of the *Code of Professional Conduct*, UKCC, 1992). Nurses also leave behind responsibility for care when their duty span is over (except in a very few units where 'pure' primary nursing operates).

For parents it is not so easy. They may be required to administer medications, give physiotherapy, dress wounds and spend many hours caring for the physical and psychological needs of the sick child and possibly other children as well. Sidey (1990) discusses the courage and commitment required by parents when they accept control. Without the commitment of parents there would be no alternative to hospital care. Generally, parents report that the advantages of home care outweigh any disadvantages (Peters and Torr, 1996), although in an evaluation of the first year of operating a new home care scheme, some parents felt that too much responsibility had been placed upon them to decide whether the child should be cared for at home or in hospital.

It is important, however, that nurses and managers do not assume that all families will be able to provide the level of skill or make the commitment to care successfully for sick children at home. Harris (1988) states that failures do occur usually because of inadequate family resources and a lack of community support. Nurses should be aware of each individual family's needs and abilities, and even if a family appears to be coping well at home they should always have the option of being able to hand back control if they feel they can no longer cope. Emotional exhaustion can add to the stress of coping for a sick child, eventually leading to the breakdown of the caring network and putting intolerable strain on family relationships. If community children's nurses are to be effective in helping families to care for sick children they should be aware of family dynamics and interactions. There may be occasions where the nurse may, with permission from the family, liaise with other professionals who can offer more appropriate support.

Hicks (1989), a social worker involved with dying children and their families, discusses the importance of communication between the social worker and the community child nurse as there is undoubtedly a role for the skills of both for many families. Health visitors and community child care nurses will need to identify clearly their roles within the family if both are involved. Professionals should be aware of their own limitations and have knowledge of the abilities and skills of others. Openness is vital because if workers are covert, conflicts will inevitably occur and the quality of care will suffer. Lask (1994) in what he describes as 'The Illness Network' identifies the importance of professionals working together as a team. It is essential, he suggests, that there are 'frequent meetings, open communication and regular reviews of the team process' (p. 998). Mutual respect and understanding are also important within a successful team approach. Where there is overlap of services, as there inevitably is, rational decisions need to be made to clarify who will do what and when. This type of approach is vital for the family caring for the child at home as it is not desirable (or cost effective) to replicate services and there is always the danger that care may be omitted as each service relies on the other to provide the care. There are many lessons to be learned from Child Protection practices (see Chapter 13) where formal and informal mechanisms exist to prevent families from 'falling through the net'.

DISCHARGE INFORMATION

Children who have been in hospital and who require continuing care at home are in a vulnerable position, regardless of whether the care is long or short term. Any period of hospitalization causes disruption of routines and anxieties for both the child and the family. Sleath (1994) highlights the need for parents to be given clear instructions and advice. It is not sufficient to give verbal advice just as the family is about to leave the ward. Discharge planning should begin from the time of admission (RCN, 1990) and may involve social workers, psychologists and other families who have experience of caring for a sick child at home which involves similar caring skills.

A study by MacDonald (1988) looked at what information mothers wanted when their children were discharged from hospital by interviewing 80 mothers. The results of the study showed that 18 mothers wanted clearer explanations, 36 wanted more information about the continuing care of the child and 24 would have liked to have a home visit. This study also showed that some mothers could not remember receiving discharge information and some had difficulty in understanding information. Ling (1996) also found that families required clarification of advice following day surgery. Nurses should ensure that they do not give too much information to parents at one time, although this is clearly difficult to avoid when children are admitted very briefly. It is also worth noting that there are factors such as anxiety and fatigue which can affect attention. In light of this it is hardly surprising that families receiving information in the midst of a busy children's ward are likely to forget some of what is said. Giving written information to back up verbal instructions is likely to help families remember what has been discussed and nurses should ensure that families have understood and remembered what they need to know.

It is important that if parents or children are expected to carry out care, the nurse should ensure that they are competent to do so. Sidey (1990) writes that, in her experience, if teaching, counselling and support are needed it is preferable that they should be carried out in the home. Obviously this is not always a viable proposition unless community child care nurses are available. Fradd (1990) discusses how parents can be invited to special workshops where they are taught skills and awarded a certificate when they become competent. Handing back control to parents has required a great deal of discussion between nurses, pharmacists, doctors and legal advisers. Fradd has found, for example, that parents are very successful at giving medication to their children (1990, p. 6):

> ...*parents take the responsibility handed to them very seriously. They have a vested interest in ensuring that the right dose of the right medicine is given at the right time.*

Dimond (1996) discusses the legal implications of parents or a child carrying out nursing care and emphasizes the importance of documenting what care is to be given by whom. As well as reviewing how parents are coping, it is also important to negotiate what level of support is required and how often respite periods are required by either the family or the child. For example, one innovative paediatric renal unit offers a 'baby sitting' service for parents caring for children with chronic renal disease and their siblings giving parents regular respite. It must again be emphasized that parents should always maintain the option of handing back control if they feel they cannot cope. If they do, then they should not be judged or made to feel incompetent. The parents should be given the opportunity to discuss their anxieties and a plan negotiated with them for future involvement.

◄ In practice

- Nurses who are involved in the discharge of children from hospital should ensure that advice to parents and children has been understood and is in a written form that can be understood.
- Community child-care nursing teams which offer 24 hour care are vital if day surgery and early discharge are to be offered as viable alternatives to hospital care.
- Health care professionals must develop effective communication networks so that the needs of the sick child and family are fully met at all times.
- If community children's nurses are visiting children, other professions (especially those with previous knowledge of the family) will have a continuing contribution to care. It is important that professionals do not concentrate only on the physical needs of the child.
- Managers need to be aware of the legal implications of being 'partners in care' with children and families.
- Parents and sick children should always retain the right to hand back responsibility to health care professionals if they can no longer cope with care.

REFERENCES

Action for Sick Children (1984) *NAWCH Charter for Children in Hospital*, NAWCH, London.

Atwell, J. and Gow, M. (1985) Paediatric trained district nurses in the community: expensive luxury or economic necessity? *British Medical Journal*, **291**, 227–9.

Audit Commission (1993) *Children First*, Audit Commission, London.

Bishop, J., Anderson, A. and McCulloch, J. (1994) Hospital at Home: a Critical Analysis. *Paediatric Nursing*, **6**(6), 13–15.

Bluebond-Langer, M. (1989) Worlds of dying children and their well siblings. *Death Studies* **13**, 1–16.

Bowlby, J. (1951) *Maternal Care and Mental Health*, World Health Organization, Geneva.

Brykczynska, G. (1987) Ethical issues in paediatric nursing. *Nursing* Series 3(23), 862–4.

Court, S.D.M. (1976) *Fit for the Future: Report of the Committee on Child Health Services,* HMSO, London.

Cowen, L., Mok, J., Corey, M., MacMillan, H., Simmons, R. and Levison, H. (1986) Psychologic adjustment of the family with a member who has cystic fibrosis. *Pediatrics,* 77(5), 745–53.

Delight, E. and Goodall, J. (1988) Babies with spina bifida treated without surgery: parents' views on home versus hospital care. *British Medical Journal,* 297, 1230–33.

Department of Health (1991) *The Welfare of Children and Young People in Hospital,* Department of Health, London.

Department of Health (1996) *Child Health in the Community: a Guide to Good Practice,* Department of Health, London.

Dimond, B. (1996) *The Legal Aspects of Child Health Care,* Mosby, London.

Doyle, B. (1987) 'I wish you were dead'. *Nursing Times,* 83(45), 44–6.

Dunn, J. (1988) Connections between Relationships: implications of research on mothers and siblings, in *Relationships Within Families: Mutual Influences,* (eds R. Hinde and J. Stevenson-Hinde), Oxford University Press, Oxford.

Dunn, J. and Kendrick, C. (1982) Temperamental differences, family relationships, and young children's response to change within the family, in *Temperamental differences in infants and young children,* CIBA Foundation Symposium, Pitman, London.

Fradd, E. (1990) Sharing accountability. *Paediatric Nursing,* 2(3), 6–8.

Glasper, A., Gow, M. and Yerrell, P. (1989) A family friend. *Nursing Times,* 85(4), 63–5.

Gould, C. (1996) Multiple Partnerships in the Community. *Paediatric Nursing,* 8(8), 28–30.

Harris, P. (1988) Sometimes pediatric home care doesn't work. *American Journal of Nursing,* 88(6), 851–4.

Hicks, A. (1989) Professional respect. *Community Care* 748, 14–15.

Kelly, P.J., Taylor, C. and Tatman, M.A. (1994/5) Hospital Outreach or Community Nursing? *Child Health,* 2(4), 160–3.

Kitson, A., Atkinson, B. and Ferguson, B. (1987) Specialist delivery of care. *Nursing Times,* 83(19), 36–40.

Kohler, J.A. and Radford, M. (1989) The dying child, in *Psychological Management of the Physically Ill,* (eds J.H. Lacey and T. Burns), Churchill Livingstone, Edinburgh.

Langlands, T. and McDonagh, L. (1995) The Pathways to Specialism. *Paediatric Nursing,* 7(8), 6–7.

Lask, B. (1994) Paediatric Liaison Work, in *Child and Adolescent Psychiatry: Modern Approaches,* 3rd edn, (eds M. Rutter, E. Taylor and L. Hersov), Blackwell Science, Oxford.

Lauer, M., Mulhern, R., Wallskog, J. and Camitta, B. (1983) A comparison study of parental adaptation following a child's death at home or in hospital. *Pediatrics,* 71(1)7, 107–12.

Lefebvre, F. and Bard, H. (1983) Montreal Canada: early discharge of preterm infants, in *Parent–Baby Attachment in Premature Infants,* (eds J.A. Davis, M.P.M. Richards and N.R.C. Robertson), Croom Helm, London.

Ling, J. (1996) Day Case Provision in a District General Hospital. *Paediatric Nursing,* 8(6), 25–8.

MacDonald, M. (1988) Children discharged from hospital – what mothers want to know. *Nursing Times*, **84**(16), 63.

Marland, J. (1994) Back Where they Belong: caring for sick children at home. *Child Health*, June/July, 40–2.

McGowan, H. (1994) Siblings and Death: Perspectives and Perception. *Paediatric Nursing*, **6**(5), 10–13.

Paediatric Nursing News (1995) PCN Shortage Stops Home Care for Sick Children. Paediatric Nursing, **6**(3), 6.

Parmelee, H. (1989) The child's physical health and the development of relationships, in *Relationship Disturbances in Early Childhood*, (eds A.J. Sameroff and R.N. Emde), Basic Books Inc, New York.

Peters, S. and Torr, G. (1996) Paediatric Hospital at Home: the first year. *Paediatric Nursing*, **8**(5), 20–3.

Platt, H. (1959) *The Welfare of Children in Hospital: Report of the Committee on Child Health Services*, HMSO, London.

Robertson, J. and Robertson, J. (1989) *Separation and the Very Young*, Free Association Press, London.

Royal College of Nursing (1990) *Standards of Care for Paediatric Nursing*, RCN, London.

Sidey, A. (1990) Co-operation in care. *Paediatric Nursing*, **2**(3), 10–12.

Sleath, K. (1994) Home Oxygenation, in *Neonatal Nursing* (eds D. Crawford and H. Morris), Chapman and Hall, London.

Strehlow, M.S. (1987) *Nursing in Educational Settings*, Harper and Row, London.

Tatman, M.A. and Woodroffe, C. (1993) Paediatric Homecare in the UK. *Archives of Disease in Childhood*, **69**, 677–8.

Tew, M. (1994) Infant Statistics, in *Neonatal Nursing* (eds D. Crawford and L. Morrison), Chapman and Hall, London.

UKCC (1992) *Code of Professional Conduct for the Nurse, Midwife and Health Visitor*, 2nd edn, UKCC, London.

UKCC (1994) *The Future of Professional Practice – the Council's Standards for Education and Practice following Registration*, UKCC, London.

UKCC (1986) *Project 2000: A New Preparation for Practice*, UKCC, London.

Whiting, M. (1989) Home truths. *Nursing Times*, **85**(14), 74–5.

To the best of our knowledge, there are no complete, comprehensive texts published as yet which discuss community children's nursing care. We would therefore refer readers to the reference list above which gives a number of journal references which will be helpful to the reader.

FURTHER READING

PART THREE

SOME SPECIAL CONSIDERATIONS

12

We have repeatedly emphasized the role of research evident in guiding nursing practice, with the ultimate aim of promoting optimal physiological and psychological functioning in individuals. It is therefore particularly disappointing to find that the research basis for nursing care of children with chronic conditions is still far from strong. It is to be hoped that this state of affairs will change, since the numbers of children suffering from long term illness is increasing. This is due mainly to improvements in medical care which have led to the survival of children who, in the past, would have died. One of the problems with research in this area arises from the vagueness of the term 'chronic illness', which not only makes interpretation of research problematic, but also leads to inconsistent decisions about where children are treated.

WHAT IS CHRONIC ILLNESS?

According to Thomas (1987, p. 5) chronic illness is:

> *any anatomical or physiological impairment that interferes with the individual's ability to function fully in the environment... The individuals' prognosis varies between a normal lifespan and unpredictable early death.*

It becomes immediately apparent that this definition allows inclusion of a wide range of conditions with an equally wide range of physical and psychological implications. One difficulty, however, when looking at research in this field is that most of the research has been undertaken with clinical samples investigating specific illnesses and conditions. There is little research which has made comparisons across illness groups which leads to problems when discussing evidence based care (Howe *et al.*, 1993). It is therefore possible to discuss, for example, the psychological implications of cystic fibrosis or epilepsy, but drawing conclusions and making generalizations about chronic illness *per se* is problematic. The term 'illness' is, in any case, often not appropriate to a chronic condition, yet its frequent use has important implications for children who may find activities, which have nothing to do with their condition, are restricted. For example, Anderson (1981) found that children with certain chronic conditions were restricted from mixing with other children even though their parents claimed to be treating them as 'normal'. For the purpose of this chapter then, chronic illness is viewed in 'functional' terms, that is in terms of its effects on the lives of children and families rather than in terms of aetiology or disease classification.

This kind of approach is implied by Perrin and Maclean (1988) who emphasize that a handicap should only refer to the consequences of a particular disability in relation to specific goals. Such an approach allows us to include handicap under the overall heading of chronic conditions although we agree with Birchenall (1995) who suggests that the term 'handicap' has what she describes as a 'socially negative value base' (p. 126). The term 'disabled' is probably no less undesirable but is in line, at least, with current practices. For both disabled children and children with other chronic conditions, there will be a range of impairment from severe to minimal and a range in prognosis from extremely poor to good, with correspondingly varied effects on development and quality of life. Constraints of space preclude detailed discussion of particular long term conditions in this chapter, and we would encourage nurses caring for children with chronic disorders to read more specific literature, perhaps using the information here as a guiding framework, and as evidence that many of the difficulties associated with chronic conditions will apply to all patients and their families, regardless of the nature of the disorder.

The nursing role

Some chronic conditions may remain under control through dietary or drug regimens, enabling the individual to reach maturity and old age with few limitations. Others will be progressive, leading to deterioration and death within months or years. Some will affect growth and development in physical terms, but leave mental functioning relatively unaffected; in other cases the reverse will be true. For the nurse, this may involve helping people to develop their (or their children's) potential, or it may mean the much sadder task of helping them come to terms with increasing limitations and disability, and possible death.

However chronic illness is conceptualized, a number of factors make the nurse's role particularly complex. Many nurses complete their training in acute settings and are likely to view any illness in terms which may only be appropriate to short term illness. Secondly, a classic piece of research by Stockwell (1972) has alerted us to the risk of unpopularity of patients who stay in hospital longer than three months (in this case adult patients), or who have some kind of condition which is felt should be treated in a different ward. It is not uncommon to hear nurses and doctors referring to chronically ill patients as 'blocking' acute beds and therefore preventing the admission of other patients.

Foster *et al.* (1989) discuss the difficulties for nurses of caring for children with chronic conditions in a setting primarily designed for acute care. Their concern introduces a major theme of this chapter, that chronic illness occurs in a long term social context, which has implications not only for nurses but for the families of patients. The nurse's role will involve families to a much greater extent in chronic illness than in acute nursing, consequently nurses will need to be informed of the effects on children and families of chronic illness. They also need to be informed of the potential stresses upon themselves of nursing chronically ill children. Blechar Gibbons and Boren (1985) discuss the conflict faced by certain paediatric nurses when caring for chronically and seriously ill children. Effective management of stress is of the utmost importance. They emphasize that the quality of care depends as much upon the psychological state of nurses as their technical expertise. This problem is more acute for nurses working in settings which group together chronically ill children, for example, nurses working on oncology wards.

FAMILY CONSEQUENCES OF CHRONIC ILLNESS

In this section, research studies are presented that suggest that families can be overlooked in the medical organization of care for the chronically sick child. Chronically ill children and their families typically experience many kinds of consequences which their healthy or 'normal' peers do not, for example:

1. repeated visits to doctors, clinics, wards or hospital departments for check-ups and therapies;
2. long term drug regimens, perhaps with unpleasant side effects;
3. chronic or continual episodes of pain, or other discomfort;
4. repeated separations from family, friends and school;
5. restrictions in activities, perhaps leading to isolation;
6. rigid or closely monitored diets;
7. constantly changing faces among caregivers; and
8. sometimes, threat of death.

Additionally, children may experience changes in the response of others to them. Parents may be unable to avoid feelings of grief and distress, and pretend that life goes on as normal (Hornby, 1991). Alternatively, they may be overprotective (Kessner Austin and McDermott, 1988; Hurst, 1996), or refuse to accept that their child cannot be cured (Foster *et al.*, 1989). Teachers may think that education is not necessary since the child has no future anyway (Lansdown and Goldman, 1988) and both parents and teachers may alter their expectations of the child because of the existence of a chronic condition, rather than because of any actual change in the child's intellectual ability. Friends may be lost through lack of contact. Hurst (1996), suggests that children may have grown up 'in the context of stereotyping that renders them passive and infantile' (p. 2). Their families may well have treated them differently from their siblings, and they may well not know how to play their part within the family. Hurst claims that over-protectiveness itself is 'an added disability' for the disabled. They may also find it difficult to attend school either through illness or hospitalization. The point here is that there is a danger of emphasizing the disability of the child rather than the child's abilities and whilst it is important to recognize the difference that chronic illness can make to the life of a child, the child and family have, according to Birchenall (1995) the right to 'an ordinary life' which emphasizes ability.

Hall (1987, p. 726) further emphasizes the need to see the child as part of the family:

> To view the child as intrinsically part of a family unit is to open the way to considering how that unit will function... The provision of support may then be oriented towards the unit rather than the individual.

This is extremely important since a number of studies have shown how family functioning can mediate the adverse effects of illness (Sloper and While, 1996; Beresford, 1994; Varni *et al.*, 1996).

CHRONIC ILLNESS AND CHILD DEVELOPMENT

It seems inevitable that the kinds of experience listed above will have some effect on a child's development. In earlier chapters, for instance, we showed that children develop largely through predictable stages, such as those described by Piaget (Chapter 4). Subsequent stages are seen to be dependent upon the achievement of earlier ones. Infants and children need to interact with and experience their environment in order to understand it and make predictions about it. Although there is an order to development, children progress at different rates, so two children of the same age may not demonstrate the same abilities.

Perrin and Gerrity (1984) have written a detailed paper discussing the development of children with chronic illness, beginning with the fact that children vary in developmental progress and that these variations occur because of variations in the child or in the environment, or both. Chronic conditions in childhood may therefore be expected to modify development because (p. 19):

> The illness affects the child's interactions with the physical and social environment in which he or she lives, and aspects of the child's environment, such as parents, peers, or school systems, are altered as a result of the illness.

They go on to provide a comprehensive discussion of normal child development and the effects chronic illness may have at any particular stage. It should be emphasized here that these are only suggestions as to potential causes of developmental delay. Perrin and Gerrity (1984) do not provide empirical evidence for all the possible effects, but merely present them as 'potential interferences with normal development imposed by chronic illness', and emphasize (p. 31) that:

> Optimal health care of these children depends on a knowledge of the risks to normal development that are regularly faced by these children at each stage of their development.

For example, immobility in infancy can prevent interaction with objects in the environment (see also Recker Baumann (1992) for details of two interesting case studies which look at children with loss of mobility). Various symptoms of illness can lead parents to doubt their ability to rear children, or many parents may use a baby's ability to feed and grow successfully as an indicator of their success as parents. A sick baby may not feed well, and may grow more slowly. Parents' feelings of inadequacy may affect their relationship with their child, and this can in turn create difficulties in terms of social development. As the baby becomes a toddler, increased motor and sensory skills allow various activities such as choosing clothes and foods, toileting skills, and more complex social interaction. Illness at this stage can delay autonomy and control, and associated treatments such as drugs which induce drowsiness will affect the child's ability to explore. Perrin and Gerrity (1984) point out the difficulties for parents in encouraging independence and normal development when it is they who must also enforce any restrictions required as a part of treatment.

In Chapter 2, we described how 1 year old infants react to strangers in the presence or absence of their parent, and chronically ill children of 2 to 3 years old may act in a similar way. Perrin and Gerrity describe ill toddlers as being more than usually tentative in their approach to new situations, and requiring more reassurance from adults than healthy toddlers. Krulik (1980) cites evidence that children with cystic fibrosis see themselves as younger than they are, dependent and inadequate, although it is interesting that Simmons *et al.* (1985) did not confirm these findings in their study of older children with cystic fibrosis.

It is easy to see how the side effects of drugs, pain and isolation from peers, family or friends may affect a child's development. Some of the goals which children of this age might normally achieve in running, climbing, jumping, writing, painting or music may be unattainable for the chronically ill child. In addition, Anderson (1981) has shown that parents may reinforce a 'generalized handicap' view of the child, by preventing the child from associating with peers in case of injury or minor illness, and by encouraging the pursuit of more solitary and more adult pen and paper skills, puzzles or conversation. Thus, the illness alone may not account for developmental underachievement. It may be that parents in fact inadvertently reduce their expectations of a child's performance at home and at school, not because of any lack of ability, but because of their perceptions of their child being ill.

McConachie and Jaffa (1996) have written a less detailed description of the effects of chronic illness on adolescent development and found that these sorts of difficulties tend to persist as the child grows older. They discuss four potential problem areas; increased vulnerability; delayed maturity; formation of identity; and emotional or behavioural difficulties. Pivotal to the development of problems they suggest is a lack of independence and opportunities to make decisions. If adolescents are to become partners in decision-making, then we cannot expect them to suddenly take on this role if they have rarely had the opportunity to practise.

Eiser (1982) cites a number of studies showing that children with a chronic illness are very often behind their healthy peers in academic achievements such as reading. Again there are a number of possible reasons for this. For example, it could be due to missed schooling arising from susceptibility to minor illness or hospital stays and check-ups, or medication could lead a child to function constantly under par or affect a child's ability directly. Eiser quotes evidence that certain treatments (such as phenytoin prescribed for epilepsy, and methotrexate and radiation therapy) are associated with reduced intellectual functioning. Additionally, teachers, like parents, may expect less of the chronically ill child who may then come to accept lower standards of achievement and make less effort.

The discussion so far in this section has been related to how development may be affected by the existence of a chronic condition. But the relationship between chronic illness and development is two-way; developmental level is also likely to affect a child's reaction to chronic illness. Chapter 4 shows how the significance of a chronic illness can become particularly worrying for adolescents, who can imagine destructive disease processes going on in the body, as well as realising the consequences in terms of future career and quality of life. Beales (1983) notes that it is important for nurses to be aware of this. It is tempting to chide an older child with comparatively mild disability who shows more distress than a younger, more severely ill patient. Beales writes:

> *The nature of a child's reaction to his condition is not simply a reflection of how brave or cowardly he happens to be. Proper understanding and management of children with chronic, disabling illnesses requires an appreciation of how the illness looks from the patient's point of view.*

Because an older child interprets pain as indicating sinister unseen damage, his or her attention will be focussed more sharply on it. Beales cites his own evidence that confirms that juvenile arthritis patients in the 12–17 age group do generally experience more severe joint pain than patients aged 6–11 years. The work of Beales and the evidence cited in Chapter 4 of this book suggest that a child's stage of development contributes to reaction to illness. Having a chronic illness clearly affects a child's achievements in various direct and indirect ways, which in turn affects development, which subsequently affects reaction to illness. The *nature* of the chronic illness does not appear to be a crucial factor in influencing this cycle (Garrison *et al*, 1990), but the role of the family does, and it is to this that discussion now turns.

IMPLICATIONS OF CHRONIC ILLNESS FOR FAMILY LIFE

Some families describe coming to terms *together* with having a sick member as a positive and beneficial experience (Parmelee, 1989; Trite, 1995). However, the literature tends to focus more on the source of stress for families, which can result in divorce, depression and psychosomatic symptoms. Brisette *et al.* (1988), in a small scale study of the effects of advanced cystic fibrosis, confirmed these symptoms with over half of the parents being divorced or experiencing marital problems and over half needing psychiatric help. Not all studies support these findings however, and there are many variables which could account for the differences such as marital relationship prior to having the ill child, social class and possibly age. Gath and Gumley (1987), for example, in their study of families with a child with Down's syndrome, did not find such adverse effects. It is clearly difficult to make sense of these findings and they may just reflect the view of Trite (1995) who suggests that adjustment by the family is not connected to the diagnosis but by a number of variables including those we have mentioned above. Trite writes:

> *having a disabled child in the family will constitute a prolonged stressor for some parents. It will require extraordinary psychological adjustment for these parents and, in some instances, require a major reorganization in the family system. For other parents, it will not be perceived as a particularly threatening or challenging circumstance, but as a natural occurrence in the life of the family which is met by smooth accommodation and seen as requiring modest adjustment (p. 1225).*

More recently however the focus of much of the literature has moved away from investigating stressors and their adverse effects towards exploring how families cope. As we mentioned earlier it is important that we view children as individuals with individual needs regardless of their medical diagnosis. Families, too, do not face chronic illness in a standardized way and there is evidence to suggest the way in which families cope with stress is as important as the source of stress because coping affects appraisal of an event and determines how an event will be dealt with. For example, Beresford (1994) discusses a number of personal coping resources which can influence how families cope with caring for a disabled child. These include the physical health of the other members of the family, beliefs, ideologies (including how flexible the family is and spiritual/religious beliefs), the personality of the family, issues surrounding control, previous coping experiences and parenting skills.

Much of the research concerning the implications of chronic illness on the family relates to stress experienced during hospitalizations, or as a result of repeated visits to hospital. Hayes and Knox (1984) carried out a qualitative study on parents of children with long term disabilities, including cancer. All parents found repeated hospitalization particularly demanding, reporting that their own lives and their whole family life revolved around the ill child's periods in hospital. Eiser (1990) emphasizes that the impact on a happy marriage is not favourable, particularly since the major burden of care and responsibility very often falls on one parent – usually, but not always, the mother. It is important that nurses attempt to include both parents in care, as Eiser emphasizes that the father can greatly facilitate the adjustment of both the child and the mother. Clearly, single parent families without the support of friends or family may need additional health care support (Beresford, 1994).

Predictably, from our discussions throughout this section of the book, there are many examples in the literature of parents who found lack of information a major source of stress (e.g. Hayes and Knox, 1984; Coombes, 1995). Hayes and Knox (1984) reported one mother who stated that it was not until she had a full understanding of the disease and its implications that she could do anything about it. Another mother's comments (on p. 338) reflect a point made in Chapter 7, that parents can do nothing towards preparation if they have no information themselves:

> *How can I do anything when I don't know what's going on? ... It's that unknown – if only I could prepare him for it.*

Hayes and Knox conclude on this point 'without exception, parents in the study emphasized the importance of clear, honest, open communication of information, endlessly repeated if necessary'. A further study by Kanneh (1990) revealed that lack of information was a major source of stress for parents. Kanneh states how important it is to address this issue as: '... parents' doubts and fears will grow if they are not informed about the progress of their child's care and condition'. Another source of stress to parents identified by Hayes and Knox (1984, p. 337) was losing control of their child's care:

> *Parents see themselves as ultimately responsible for their child's care and need to be able to trust that the health professional is competent and cares for their child and cares about them as a family.*

This feeling of responsibility that parents have can lead to feelings of guilt if they need some relief from constantly caring for their chronically ill child. Attention may focus so completely on their child that the needs of the parents are neither recognized nor met. Nielson (1990) writes a poignant account of her experiences as a mother of a chronically ill baby which suggests that nurses may unwittingly reinforce this problem. Parents may at times feel unable to cope physically or psychologically with the responsibility of caring. When Nielson felt she could no longer feed her ill son because of the 'energy and skill' required she writes that the nurses 'thought I was rejecting my baby'. It is important that nurses are perceptive to parental needs and respect their wishes about both the level of participation and the time they need for themselves without making parents feel guilty, inadequate or as Nielson writes 'unstable'. Respite care for parents can certainly be a positive experience for parents and should be seen as a planned necessity rather than as a measure to be taken when parents can no longer cope. Beresford (1994) suggests that respite care can be a preventive strategy to help parents avoid some of the stresses of continuous care and describes schemes including the 'Link Family Scheme' in which the family of the disabled child are linked with another family with no disabled children (a similar philosophy to *PHAB*). The family participates in aspects of caring for the disabled child and is able to give the parents of the disabled child a few precious hours of space. We described earlier a similar scheme which is offered by nurses in a renal unit.

These types of scheme are an important source of social support for families in terms of preventing the long term effects on parents which can be serious if parental needs are not considered. Carr (1988) in her study of families with a child with Down's syndrome found that their physical and psychological wellbeing was frequently affected. Mothers tended to have higher morbidity than other family members. Hayes and Knox's (1984) major finding was that parents see their role in the hospitalized child's care differently from the health professionals. They suggest that much parental stress is attributable to the 'space' between health workers' understanding of parents' experience and the parents' own comprehension, and feel that if nurses understood parents' views better, more effective nursing care could be developed. It is clear, and Hayes and Knox acknowledge this, that this is an area where further research is required before any specific suggestions can be put forward.

Sibling effects

It is not just parents who are affected by a child's chronic illness, but siblings too. In Chapter 3 we discussed the effect on siblings of the hospitalization of an ill brother or sister, and for a chronically ill child's siblings this is going to be particularly disruptive. A study by Stewart *et al.* (1992) related to this problem. They studied the psychosocial functioning of 10 siblings of children with chronic life threatening illness and found marked levels of distress in some siblings when matched with healthy controls. Part of the difficulties for siblings related to the loss of social life experienced by their mothers and difficulty in their relationships with their fathers who to some extent excluded themselves from the family.

A study by Craft and Wyatt (1986) studied a group of siblings of children hospitalized for various conditions including chronic illness. They found that siblings experienced difficulty in sleeping and increased nervousness. They did not find, surprisingly, that if siblings were allowed more contact with the ill child and parents that changes in feelings and behaviour were any less. It was, however, a relatively small study and there is clearly a need for further research in this field, particularly research which includes healthy controls, such as in the study by Stewart *et al.* (1992). In a review of the relatively few studies on siblings resulting from the existence of a chronically ill brother or sister, Ferrari (1984) notes the lack of control groups for each study. Hence, although there is evidence of behavioural problems, maladjustment and resentment in the siblings, it is difficult to determine the degree to which the incidence was higher than the norm for healthy families. Where control families have been used, sibling maladjustment is still reported but the rates are lower than in the uncontrolled studies. Indeed, Breslau *et al.* (1981) in a large study using controls found that the siblings of chronically ill children did not have a significantly higher *overall* rate of emotional and behavioural problems than the siblings of healthy children. They only found significant differences in three of the seven areas studied, which were 'mentation problems', 'fighting' and 'delin-quency'. Another very interesting finding of the study related to gender and the birth order of the sibling in relation to the ill child. Younger male siblings and older female siblings had more problems than older males and younger females. It does appear, therefore, that to a varying degree, the existence of a chronically ill child in the family may have a negative effect on the psychological development of healthy brothers and sisters.

Ferrari's own research (1984), with 48 children representing three points along a continuum of disability (ranging from highly visible and disabling chronic conditions to healthy), failed to support the view that siblings of chronically ill children are *uniformly* at greater risk of psycho-social impairment than siblings of healthy children. Sibling adjustment depended in part on the adjustment of others in the child's environment, especially the child's mother. Ferrari concludes (p. 474): 'Following from this, therapeutic approaches should emphasize the involvement of all family members'. He also draws attention to the variability in the effects he found. It is clear from his work that no clear pattern of distur-bance in siblings emerges, even where families were coping with the same illness, which he suggests:

> *Strongly argues for the need for individualized assessment and treatment of families where coping with the onset of chronic illness in one of its members may be causing a great deal of hardship.*

Lansdown and Goldman (1988) have pointed out that siblings need to be, and often are, very knowledgeable about the illness, treatment and prognosis although they warn against giving the sibling more infor-mation than the ill child. Siblings will often be well integrated into family routines which may appear casual but which actually reflect a system uniquely adapted by the family to the individual sick child's need as well as those of the family as a whole. This kind of family organi-zation, which may function efficiently in the community, can be badly disrupted by hospitalization, if health professionals do not appreciate the differences between the needs of acutely ill children and the established patterns of care in some families with chronically ill children. In cases where the family are generally coping well with the demands of the child's life, parents will often have more knowledge and expertise than the nurses, and expect to be involved in decision-making and care planning. It is important that nursing staff are aware of the child's individual goals and do not undermine the achievements of parents or other professionals. It is likely that other health workers will be involved with the child, for example, speech and language therapists, social workers, physiotherapists, community nurses and doctors. A study by Alcock and Mahoney (1990) showed that most parents had met more than 27 professionals involved in the care of their child. Knowledge of goals and coordination of care is vital in order to reduce parental anxiety when children are hospitalized. Similarly, the reason for hospitalization may threaten their established coping patterns, as when it represents a deterioration in a fatal condition. We cannot view the adjustments and adaptations the whole families are able to make as static and permanent achievements. These processes are dynamic, and modify in response to environmental, social and cognitive pressures. It is important for nurses to keep alert to factors which may pose threats to established methods of coping, and they need to work with families in reviewing and updating knowledge about their needs.

Family coping

Various suggestions emerge from research studies for improving family coping. Typical examples include involving more than just the primary caregiver in the planning and giving of care. The other parent, siblings and grandparents could be involved to spread responsibility and pressure. Another suggestion concerns giving accurate information to all concerned and repeating it as often as necessary. Several people suggest providing opportunities for prolonged discussion and the opportunity to show feelings. Nurses are encouraged to learn their role with each child from the people who usually give the care, and to design care plans which reflect the unusual nature of chronic illness rather than trying to use materials more suited to acute admissions. The same applies to routines and procedures, which in acute settings may be inappropriately organized for chronically ill children.

An important recent development in research on children with chronic illness is a concentration on 'normalization'. Normalization promotes optimum development, a 'normal lifestyle within a normal framework for effective living' (Brown, 1991). There is a prevailing desire for 'normalcy' in Western society, and Brown suggests it has been frequently adopted by government services in terms of 'nomenclature' (p. 13). There is however a paradoxical situation, since restrictions on the children's lives, such as isolation from peers, regulation of the child's life by drug schedules, unusual dietary requirements and restriction on physical activities, can give the message 'you are not well, you are different', whereas parents are communicating the conflicting message 'you are well, you are normal'. What these parents do is to *minimize* the effects of chronic illness. They do this by working as a family, rather than focussing on the ill child.

Interventions at family level require that nurses understand how the family, as a unit, could modify its lifestyle to 'normalize' the ill child's life. Anderson (1981) suggests that health teaching of this kind could be of particular value when dietary patterns need to be changed and exercise programmes implemented, and adds that this will reduce labelling the patient as 'sick', and has the bonus of instituting a healthier lifestyle for all family members. There are various 'normalizing' tactics which can be adopted such as introducing a particular diet (e.g. a fat-free one) on the whole family, or sending a wheat free cookbook to a cookery class at school so that the whole class can cook and eat the appropriate food. Physiotherapy exercises can be done not just by the child but by the child's friends and other members of the family. If the child requires medication, such as vitamin pills, the whole family can take them or if the child has to take different pills at a particular time (e.g. breakfast time) the rest of the family can take vitamins so that the whole family is taking medication albeit of a different type. Anderson (1981) concludes that nurses and other health professionals can use these principles to plan intervention and guide parents, teachers and others who come into contact with the chronically ill child. Another strategy for achieving normalization is reported by Holaday (1984) who writes that parents may attempt to intervene with social groups with which the child has contact in order to facilitate the child's integration with that group. An example of this would be the mother who works as a volunteer in the child's school where she can assist with the child's physical needs, thus reducing dependence on peers or teachers which may involve the child becoming stigmatized. If, however, parents intervene in most or all the social groups with which the child has inter- action the child may find it distressing when the support is no longer there. Again, it must be stressed that nurses must attempt to understand how families function as a unit if they are to gain insight into the needs of the child.

In this chapter we have discussed chronic illness in terms of its effects, which are clearly potentially stressful for the child, the family and the health care team. It is recognized that an understanding of the potential stresses can help nurses to deal sympathetically with an upset child, an exhausted parent, or a 'neglected' sibling. 'Normalizing' tactics can help reduce the impact of chronic illness on a child, but the experience of a chronically ill child in the family must still be recognized as an extremely demanding one.

In practice ➤

- Many of the implications of research presented in other chapters in this book also apply to chronically ill children. However, chronic illness occurs in a long term social context and the effect on the child and family will be exacerbated. It is important that nurses are sensitive to the stresses chronic illness brings to family life.
- On the other hand, parents may reinforce chronically ill children's views of themselves as different, and expect a lower standard of achievement. Nurses can encourage parents to treat their child in as normal a way as possible. Another way of minimizing a feeling of being different is to involve other

members of the family in diets and exercises prescribed for the ill child.

- Chronically ill children may be immobile and therefore unable to experience their environment in the way that healthy children do. This lack of stimulation can affect development, so it is worthwhile taking extra care to entertain such children in hospital. For example, provision of adapted mobile trolleys allows greater exploration and hence wider experience.

- Missing school is one of the contributory factors to lower achievement in chronically ill children. It is important therefore to recognize that teachers provide a particularly important service to these children, and that school work should be given priority in the planning of the child's day, wherever possible. In the absence of formal classes, nurses can encourage parents to keep in touch with the child's usual school and help set appropriate goals.

- Developmental level can affect a child's reaction to chronic illness. Older children may be more upset than younger ones because they understand the implications of their illness for quality of life. Nurses need to be aware of this and give time and encouragement for discussion of children's particular worries.

- Many parents of chronically ill children become frustrated and upset at the lack of information given to them. Accurate information should be freely provided both at the time of diagnosis and throughout the period of the families' contact with the hospital.

- Caring for a chronically ill child is disruptive and exhausting for parents. They may need encouragement from nursing staff to take a break, without feelings of guilt.

- Siblings can feel rejected and resentful. A warm welcome from nurses in the hospital can help them to feel included in the sick child's special world, and also serve as a gentle reminder to parents that their other children also have important needs.

- Both parents and siblings often become very knowledgeable about illness, treatments and prognosis and will often have developed efficient coping systems. It is to the benefit, therefore, of nursing staff to involve parents and older siblings in decision-making and care planning, so that each person responsible for the child's care knows about that child's individual needs and achievements.

REFERENCES

Alcock, D. and Mahoney, W. (1990) Parents of long stay children. *The Canadian Nurse*, 86(19), 21–3.

Anderson, J.M. (1981) The social construction of illness experience: families with a chronically ill child. *Journal of Advanced Nursing*, 6, 427–34.

Beales, G. (1983) The child's view of chronic illness. *Nursing Times*, 79(51), 50–1.

Beresford, B.A. (1994) Resources and Strategies: How Parents Cope with the Care of a Disabled Child. *Journal of Child Psychology and Psychiatry*, 35(1), 171–209.

Birchenall, M. (1995) Disability: An Issue for the Growing Child, in *Childhood to Adolescence: Caring for Health*, (ed. A. Fatchett), Baillière Tindall, London.

Blechar Gibbons, M. and Boren, H. (1985) Stress reduction: a spectrum of strategies in pediatric oncology nursing. *Nursing Clinics of North America*, 20(1), 83–103.

Breslau, N., Weitzman, M. and Messenger, K. (1981) Psychologic functioning of siblings of disabled children. *Pediatrics*, 67(3), 344–53.

Brisette, S., Zinman, R. and Reidy, M. (1988) Disclosure of psychosocial concerns of young adults with advanced cystic fibrosis by a nurse home visiting program. *International Journal of Nursing Studies*, 25(1),67–72.

Brown, R.I. (1991) Changing Concepts of Disability, in *Early Intervention Studies for Young Children with Special Needs*, (eds D. Mitchell and R.I. Brown), Chapman and Hall, London.

Carr, J. (1988) 6 weeks to 21 years: a longitudinal study of children with Down's Syndrome and their families. *Journal of Child Psychology and Psychiatry*, 29(4), 407–31.

Coombes, R. (1995) From Parent to Expert. *Child Health*, 2(6), 237–40.

Craft, M. and Wyatt, N. (1986) Effect of visitation upon siblings of hospitalized children. *Maternal–Child Nursing Journal*, 15(1), 47–59.

Eiser, C. (1982) The effects of chronic illness on children and their families, in *Social Psychology and Behavioural Medicine*, (ed. J.R. Eiser), John Wiley, Chichester.

Eiser, C. (1990) Psychological effects of chronic disease. *Journal of Child Psychology and Psychiatry*, 31(1), 85–98.

Ferrari, M. (1984) Chronic illness: psychosocial effects on siblings. *Journal of Child Psychology and Psychiatry*, 25, 459–76.

Foster, R., Hunsberger, M. and Anderson, J. (1989) *Family Centred Nursing Care of Children*, T.B. Saunders, Philadelphia.

Garrison, W.T., Biggs, D. and Williams, K. (1990) Temperament characteristics and clinical outcomes in young children with diabetes mellitus. *Journal of Child Psychology and Psychiatry*, 31(7), 1079–88.

Gath, A. and Gumley, D. (1987) Retarded children and their siblings. *Journal of Child Psychology and Psychiatry*, 28(5), 715–30.

Hall, D. (1987) Social and psychological care before and during hospitalisation. *Social Science Medicine*, 25(6), 721–32.

Hayes, V.E. and Knox, J.E. (1984) The experience of stress in parents of children hospitalized with long term disabilities. *Journal of Advanced Nursing*, 9, 333–41.

Holaday, B. (1984) Challenges of rearing a chronically ill child: caring and coping. *Nursing Clinics of North America*, 19(2), 361–9.

Hornby, G. (1991) Parent Involvement, in *Early Intervention Studies for Young Children with Special Needs*, (eds D. Mitchell and R.I. Brown), Chapman and Hall, London.

Howe, G.W., Feinstein, C., Reiss, D., Molock, S. and Berger, K. (1993) Adolescent Adjustment to Chronic Physical Disorders – I: Comparing Neurological and Non Neurological Conditions. *Journal of Child Psychology and Psychiatry*, 34(7), 1153–71.

Hurst, R. (1996) A Disabled Persons' Viewpoint, in *Services for Young People with Chronic Disorders: in their transition from childhood to adult life*, (eds Z. Kurtz and A Hopkins), Royal College of Physicians, London.

Kanneh, A. (1990) The need to communicate. *Nursing Standard*, 5(5), 19–20.

Kessner Austin, J. and McDermott, N. (1988) Parental attitude and coping behaviors in families of children with epilepsy. *The American Association of Neuroscience Nursing*, 20(3), 174–9.

Krulik, T. (1980) Successful 'normalizing' tactics of parents of chronically-ill children. *Journal of Advanced Nursing*, 5, 573–8.

Lansdown, R. and Goldman, A. (1988) The psychological care of children with malignant disease. *Journal of Child Psychology and Psychiatry*, 29(5), 555–67.

McConachie, H. and Jaffa, T. (1996) Psychology of Adolescent Development, in *Services for Young People with Chronic Disorders: in their transition from childhood to adult life*, (eds Z. Kurtz and A. Hopkins), Royal College of Physicians, London.

Nielson, D. (1990) One parent's perspective. *The Canadian Nurse*, 86(19), 18–19.

Parmelee, A. (1989) The child's physical health and the development of relationships, in *Relationship Disturbances in Early Childhood*, (A.J. Sameloff and R.N. Emde), Basic Books, New York.

Perrin, E.C. and Gerrity, S.P. (1984) Development of children with a chronic illness. *Pediatric Clinics of North America*, 31, 19–31.

Perrin, J. and Maclean, W. (1988) Children with chronic illness: prevention of dysfunction. *Pediatric Clinics of North America*, 35(6), 1325–37.

Recker Baumann, D. (1992) Coping Behavior of Children Experiencing Loss of Mobility, in *Coping with Chronic Illness: Overcoming Powerlessness*, (ed. J. Fitzgerald Miller), F.A. Davis, Philadelphia.

Simmons, R.J., Corey, M., Cowen, L., Keenan, N., Robertson, J. and Levison, H. (1985) Emotional adjustments of early adolescents with cystic fibrosis. *Psychosomatic Medicine*, 47(2), 111–21.

Sloper, P. and While, D. (1996) Risk factors in the Adjustment of Children with Cancer. *Journal of Child Psychology and Psychiatry*, 37(5), 597–607.

Stewart, D.A., Stein, A., Forrest, G.C. and Clark, D.M. (1992) Psychosocial Adjustments in Siblings of Children with Chronic Life Threatening Illness. *Journal of Child Psychology and Psychiatry*, 33(4), 779–84.

Stockwell, F. (1972) *The Unpopular Patient*, RCN, London.

Thomas, R.B. (1987) Introduction and conceptual framework, in *Children with Chronic Conditions: Nursing in a Family and Community Context*, (eds M.H. Rose and R.B. Thomas), Grune and Stratton, Orlando.

Trite, B. (1995) Gender Differences in the Psychological Adjustment of Parents of Young Developmentally Disabled Children. *Journal of Child Psychology and Psychiatry*, 36(7), 1225–42.

Varni, J.W., Katz, E.R., Colegrove, R. and Dolgin, M. (1996) Family Functioning Predictors of Adjustment in Children with Newly Diagnosed Cancer: a prospective analysis. *Journal of Child Psychology and Psychiatry*, 37(3), 321–8.

FURTHER READING

Clarke, P., Kofsky, H. and Lauruol, J. (1989) *To a Different Drumbeat*, Hawthorn Press, Stroud.

A book written for parents by parents of children with special needs. This book gives nurses valuable insight into the frustrations of being a parent of special children.

Kurtz, Z. and Hopkins, A. (eds) (1996) *Services for Young People with Chronic Disorders: in their transition from childhood to adult life*. Royal College of Physicians, London.

This collection of papers is written from a number of professional viewpoints as well as from the viewpoint of service users. Whilst it particularly relates to adolescents it is apparent that many of the problems experienced by young people have their origins in childhood. It is essential reading for any nurse who works with young people with chronic illness (unusually there is even a section specifically about outpatient departments which is excellent).

IDENTIFYING AND PREVENTING CHILD ABUSE 13

Community and hospital based nurses working in the field of child health will be involved with families where it is known, or suspected, that a child or children are being abused. A knowledge of psychology relating to the prevention, detection and management of child abuse is necessary in order to be able to provide relevant and competent care. This chapter aims, therefore, to discuss the psychological nature of child abuse. Our knowledge in this field has been greatly enhanced by a number of research papers published in the 'Studies in Child Protection' series. These studies focus on a wide range of issues around the operation of the child protection system, the prevalence of abuse, the perceptions of parents and children of the child protection system and the effects of abuse on the individual children and their families.

Whilst these studies have increased the research base of child protection issues, they have raised awareness of anomalies within the operation of the system, particularly in relation to the variations which exist between local authorities in, for example, the use of the child protection register and the involvement of parents in child protection procedures. These studies have made sound, evidence based recommendations to address anomalies and we look forward to the future replication of these studies to see whether the recommendations have been followed and if they have been effective.

PSYCHOLOGICAL APPROACHES

The psychological study of child protection raises at least three broad questions, which are of particular importance to nursing. These questions are:

1. the study of person perception, that is how we make judgements about other people;
2. issues raised in attempting to predict human behaviour; and
3. the problem of implementing treatment in the management of children and parents.

Our knowledge of psychology shows how one must approach these with extreme caution and sensitivity, while realizing that the welfare of children in our care is paramount.

Perception of people

In judging what other people are like, we often have to base our decisions on relatively superficial cues. To some extent we cluster together a number of attributes in coming to a viewpoint. Stockwell (1972), for example, in her well known study, found that nurses had fairly typical stereotypes of the unpopular patient. Similar findings have been reported by Wattley and Müller (1984) in a series of practicals designed to investigate how we perceive others. These findings are of particular importance both in identifying and in predicting child abuse and neglect. On the one hand, in order to help nurses and health visitors, it is useful to have a checklist consisting of those factors which are most likely to be present in families where child abuse and neglect are prevalent and we are aware that the use of vulnerability checklists is indeed widespread among health professionals. However, to some extent, by using a checklist, one is contributing towards a stereotyped view of the abusing parent.

Predicting behaviour

There is a similar problem in attempting to predict whether, if left in a family, a particular child will be subject to further abuse. The issue here is one of evaluating whether any decision taken will be right or wrong. Unfortunately, it is only afterwards that it can be seen whether a child should have been removed from home or not.

The Butler-Sloss report (1988) discussed the dilemma of those involved in child protection. On many occasions workers have been criticized severely because they have not taken action to remove the child from the potential abuser. On the other hand in the Cleveland enquiry workers were criticized because of 'over-enthusiasm and zeal in actions taken'. Furthermore, when the decision is right to keep a family together this is rarely reported (Sharman, 1983). This issue is of particular concern to community nurses in their work with families.

There are data which provide some evidence about the likelihood of repetition of abuse but the extent to which these data are helpful in terms of decision-making is questionable. Gibbons *et al.* (1995a) compared pre-school children placed on child protection registers for physical abuse 10 years after the original notification on the register with a sample of 'normal children' (defined as children of the same age and sex who lived nearby and attended the same school but who had never been involved in the child protection system). Whilst the main aim of their study was to investigate the long term consequences of physical abuse, the study also identified repetition of abuse. They found a total re-injury rate of 20% but recognized that this may be a low estimate. The only predictive trend of repetition (which did not reach statistical significance) was that the original perpetrator of the abuse was more likely to have been the mother. However, where the perpetrator had been the father and where the abuse was particularly serious it was likely that the child would be separated from the perpetrator either because the perpetrator left home or the child was placed in care outside the home. Therefore these data do not enable us to determine what would have happened had all the children been left at home in the same environment as that which existed at the time of the original abuse.

Two further studies found slightly higher repetition rates. Gibbons *et al.* (1995b) found a repetition rate of 31 per cent over a 26 week period following registration and Farmer and Owen (1995) a rate of 30 per cent after 20 months. These rates may reflect the current practice of keeping families together where possible, whereas in the study by Gibbons *et al.* (1995a) registration had taken place 10 years before when children were more likely to be separated from the perpetrator. Farmer and Owen's (1995) study did attempt to explore this issue and unfortunately found that of those children in their sample who were left with the abusing adult for all or at least part of the time, 43 per cent had not been safe and the system had not been effective in protecting them.

The shift towards keeping families together and attempting to work in partnership with families (Hallett, 1995) was driven by the *Children Act* (DoH, 1989) and the following guidance *Working Together Under the Children Act* (Home Office *et al.*, 1991). Thoburn *et al.* (1995) explore this issue and conclude that both professionals and families have welcomed the increased participation which extends to the formulation of the child protection plan and the facilitation of greater cooperation between families and professionals. However, in light of Farmer and Owen's (1995) findings it may be time to review the current practice or at least further explore predictors of outcome.

What is important is that community nurses try to be objective in their decision-making and do not allow external pressures, particularly from the media, to influence their judgement. This point was raised by Jackson (1989) who discusses MacLeod's observations with social work students before and after the event in Cleveland:

> *Using the same case study – a physically abused child – she found that pre Cleveland all the students elected to put the child into care; post-Cleveland they all felt that the child should remain at home.*

Managing care

The issue concerning intervention is one which has been given less consideration from a nursing perspective, and yet it is an area of extreme importance. Community nurses, particularly health visitors, are seen to be very well placed to be involved in intervention given their knowledge of the geographic area in which they work and their unique contact with individual families. Kent (1988) noted that official inquiries into the deaths of two children both called for a 'more positive approach' by health visitors. Taylor and Tilley (1989) also supported the view that health visitors should be involved in the management as well as the identification of child abuse and current research suggests that this is indeed what happens in practice (Farmer and Owen, 1995; Hallett, 1995).

On the other hand, there are negative aspects to health visitors taking a more active role where abuse is known to have taken place. The emphasis of contemporary health visiting practice is on the prevention of ill health and its consequences, health promotion and more generally on public health issues. Hallett (1995) found in her study that health visitors and their managers were anxious that they should not be used in the management of child protection where there were clear indications that social work intervention would be more appropriate. Hallett found, however, that in some cases health visitors were forced to undertake social work roles within families because of the resource position in social service departments. We would argue that this should never be to the detriment of the health visitor's relationship with the family, particularly if there is a risk that the health visitor might be denied access to the family because of the threshold of what should be essentially social worker type intervention.

Nicol (1989) indicates that abused children are actually more likely to have emotional development problems as a result of their experiences. This view is largely supported by the 10 year follow up study undertaken by Gibbons *et al.* (1995a). It is important then that the health visitor's relationship with the child and family enables them to fulfil their preventive and health promotion roles to prevent the detrimental effects of earlier abuse and detect early those adverse effects which cannot be prevented so that effective intervention can be instigated.

Occasionally, in individually defined cases as a result of the child protection plan, health visitors may take a more active role if they are perceived to be the most appropriate person to do so although a social worker will always take on the role of key worker. They may, for example, have a well established relationship with the family which gives a good basis upon which to carry out effective intervention. The point is that in managing child abused families it is important to undertake the most effective and efficient forms of treatment. Programmes of intervention should be systematically evaluated. Psychologists have particular skills in this area and it is important that they become involved with nurses in this kind of work. The involvement of health visitors in the active management of child abused families could however be detrimental to their public image (Corby, 1995). Taylor and Tilley (1989) warn that, if health visitors become more involved with child protection, it could compromise their position in the identification of other potentially abused children as parents may be reluctant to allow access to their child. Taylor and Tilley write:

> *There is thus a contradiction between open participation in child protection and those conditions which place the health visitor in an ideal position to take part in it.*

Nurses working in hospital may also find themselves involved in the identification and management of child abuse. The Butler-Sloss report (1988) highlighted many of the problems faced by nurses involved in the care of abused children. As a result of litigation by social services, suspected child abuse victims and their siblings were admitted to paediatric wards. This practice raises many issues for nurses, especially if parental access is denied. On the one hand, nurses are encouraging parental participation in care for children in hospital while on the other the Court may make that participation illegal. Our knowledge of the detrimental effects of hospitalization on children (see Chapter 7), especially when they are separated from parents, raises many questions for nurses in these situations. On the other hand, children who have suffered abuse need protection from their abuser. Clearly nurses need to have a sound understanding of the psychological needs of children and their families as well as knowledge relating to the legal and ethical issues in caring for such families.

THE NATURE OF CHILD ABUSE

It is difficult to know the extent to which children are abused by their families. It has been argued that the definition of child abuse itself rests on a moral judgement about the boundaries between legitimate discipline and cruel treatment (Parker, 1995). In 1988, for the first time, the Department of Health undertook a national survey and revealed that 40 000 children in England alone were on child protection registers (Parker, 1995) – a rate of 3.5 children per 1000 population below the age of 18 years. At this time the statistics showed that 28 per cent of the children registered were physically abused, 15 per cent were sexually abused, 13 per cent were registered because of neglect, 4 per cent for emotional abuse, 3 per cent were registered under mixed categories and 37 per cent because of 'grave concern' (Parker, 1995). Since that time, and probably due in part to the media reporting of sexual abuse in Cleveland rates for sexual abuse registrations rose to around 26 per cent in 1993. However, these data may also reflect that, after 1991 the registerable category of 'grave concern' was removed because of the suspicion that some children may have been registered as a way of gaining additional resources for the family rather than because of a genuine need to protect them from abuse. All children previously registered under this category were re-categorized at their next periodic review, meaning that the category of sexual abuse after 1991 included children who had been sexually abused or who were likely to be sexually abused. It is interesting to note however that a study by Gibbons *et al.* (1995b) found that some local authorities continue to register children under the grave concern category even though the category no longer officially exists.

Categories of child abuse

There are now four categories that can be used to place the names of children on child protection registers (Home Office *et al.*, 1991):

1. physical injury;
2. sexual abuse;
3. neglect; and
4. emotional abuse.

Physical injury refers to: *'actual or likely physical injury to a child, or failure to prevent physical injury (or suffering) to a child including deliberate poisoning, suffocation and Munchausen's syndrome by proxy'.*

Munchausen syndrome by proxy is a term used to describe children whose carer (usually the mother) invents or fabricates signs of illness which subjects the child to needless investigations (Meadow 1989). One well documented example of Munchausen's syndrome by proxy, which involved a carer (in this case a nurse rather than the mother) can be found in the *Allitt Inquiry* (Clothier *et al.*, 1994).

Sexual abuse is defined as: *'actual or likely sexual exploitation of a child or adolescent. The child may be dependant and/or developmentally immature'* (Home Office *et al.*, 1991).

Sexual abuse includes such activities as indecent acts, pornographic photography involving children, fondling and penetrative acts including incest. Hobbs and Wynne (1990) in their longitudinal study of 2883 children referred with suspected abuse, found that 16.9 per cent of physically abused children and 13.6 per cent of sexually abused children had actually suffered both forms of abuse.

As we have mentioned above, sexual abuse was brought to the attention of the media because of the events that occurred in Cleveland in the late 1980s. There is some speculation as to the actual prevalence of sexual abuse (remember that we only have data relating to children who have been *registered* and this might not accurately reflect the extent of the problem within the population). One of the *Studies in Child Protection* series (Ghate and Spencer, 1995) has explored the methodological difficulties of investigating this area and established that it would be possible to carry out prevalence studies.

Neglect, which is particularly difficult to notice, can persist for some time before being identified. It is identified by the Home Office *et al.* (1991) as: *'persistent or severe neglect of a child, or the failure to protect a child from exposure to any kind of danger, including cold or starvation, or extreme failure to carry out important aspects of care, resulting in the significant impairment of the child's health or development, including non-organic failure to thrive'.* Neglect, therefore, occurs when those who are responsible for meeting the basic needs of the child, at whatever level, fail to do so either by commission or *omission*. That is to say the harm is caused because of a failure to provide care rather than by deliberate action.

Emotional abuse nearly always coincides with physical ill treatment, but can occur as a form of abuse in itself and should only be used in terms of registration where it is the main or sole form of abuse. This might be the case when children are rejected or even terrorized. It can result in the child failing to thrive as well as bizarre behaviour patterns. Emotional abuse is defined as: *'actual or likely severe adverse effect on the emotional and behavioural development of a child caused by persistent emotional ill-treatment or rejection. All abuse involves some emotional ill-treatment. This category should be used where it is the main or sole form of abuse'* (Home Office *et al*, 1991).

It is important, however, to understand child abuse in the social context of normal family life. Most families have to deal with both direct and indirect forms of aggression, and outbursts of temper are not uncommon. One expects then, some degree of tension between parents and their children. The important question is how this anger is dealt with. Families evolve differing strategies, some successful others not, to keep their lives on an even keel. It is in those families who are unsuccessful in doing this where child abuse might occur.

Frude (1980), in an early but useful discussion into the psychological factors relating to child abuse, makes it extremely clear that it cannot be seen as a specific syndrome. Indeed, he stresses the importance of taking a broad view of the nature of child abuse and notes (p. 6) that:

> *injury deliberately inflicted on children by their parents is of many types and that the personality of the parents themselves, their social background, the circumstances in which the attack takes place and the age and personality of the child involved all vary prodigiously.*

Frude (1980) discusses the research by Gaensbauer and his colleagues which shows that, although the reactions of abused children are to some extent associated with style of mother–child interaction, there is still considerable variability in their responses. Gibbons *et al.* (1995a and b) in their 10 years follow up study of children who had been physically abused supported this view and found that even where children had been removed from perpetrators of abuse they did not significantly improve in terms of outcomes. They conclude that children may actually need help in terms of helping them to form relationships. Browne (1995) also suggests that some children may themselves 'be instrumental in some way in eliciting attack or neglect' (p. 49). That is not to say that the children are in any way to blame for the abuse or that they encourage it, but rather that the children themselves are not sterile recipients of a relationship but an integral part of it.

It is of interest that Gibbons *et al.* (1995a) also found that harmful parenting methods including physical 'punitive methods' (p. 176) were evident as often in adoptive homes as in natural families which might add further support to the idea of abused children as 'special victims' (Browne, 1995). Alternatively, it may be that some abused children have developed coping mechanisms for dealing with previous abuse which persist following adoption and which might in some way encourage harmful parenting. Gibbons *et al.* (1995a) found, however, that such harmful parenting was not apparent in foster homes, presumably because of continuing social worker involvement.

Millor (1981), an American nurse researcher, suggests that there are situational conditions and personal characteristics which are contributing factors to the way parents perceive their roles. Parental attitudes are shaped by their own experiences as children, and by community and family tolerances towards the physical punishment of children. Added to this are the parents' self-characteristics and their role expectations. Normally one expects 'normative nurturance' and 'normative discipline'.

However, where there are stressful family transactions and the child has certain characteristics which result in unacceptable kinds of behaviour, the way the parents have defined their roles can determine whether neglect or abuse results. Millor's work provides a useful framework which she suggests is helpful to the nurse researcher. Her suggestion that nurses have an important role to play in working with other professionals in this area is substantiated in this chapter. What is clear from these discussions, however, is that it is difficult to generalize too widely about the nature of abuse and the precipitating factors.

IDENTIFYING CHILD ABUSE

Nurses who are especially likely to come into contact with children who have been abused, are those working in accident and emergency departments. An interesting study conducted by Dingwall (1983a) has shown some strategies adopted in trying to detect child abuse in hospitals with accident services. The research was carried out in four English hospitals (one of which was a teaching hospital). Observational and interview data were collected and it was found that challenges were dictated towards parents on the basis of their demeanour in discussion and according to any information of an adverse nature included on their admission records. In one hospital, all child admissions from a local gypsy site were considered possible victims of maltreatment until proven otherwise. This is clearly a particularly vindictive form of stereotyping and one which could have serious consequences. Dingwall emphasizes the need to be cautious and not discourage parents from bringing in children in need of care.

The study by Dingwall (1983a) does show that the nurse, who will often spend a significant amount of time with the child, has a very important role to play in detecting abuse, especially as another finding was that the medical staff focussed much more on the nature of the injuries than on their cause. He also noted that nurses in the non-teaching hospitals tended to have more local knowledge and be better informed about families where abuse was likely. Dingwall suggests that an expensive but useful approach in detecting child abuse might be some kind of integration between accident and emergency nursing and community nursing. Taylor and Tilley (1989), in their research into health visitor involvement in child protection in two health authorities, discuss a system of close communication between field health visitors and accident and emergency staff in one of the health authorities studied. Communication is, no doubt, improved but Taylor and Tilley question the ethics of such liaison, which involves written records and communications, and which is done without the knowledge or consent of parents. However, the Department of Health and the Welsh Office (1995) clarify this issue and suggest that 'it is good practice for arrangements to be made to notify the health visitor or school nurse, as appropriate, of all visits made by children 0–16 years to the accident and emergency department' (p. 14). They also emphasize the need for accident and emergency staff to notify the GP of visits and stress the importance of not delaying when making such communications.

As we have mentioned above, accident and emergency staff are often involved in the detection of abuse on the basis of cues such as frequent attendance or implausibility and inconsistent explanations in relationship to the injury (DoH/Welsh Office, 1995). Sometimes, however, the suspicion of abuse is not based upon such tangible evidence but rather because nurses 'feel' that something is not quite right. In either case, it is important that nurses communicate their suspicions to a senior colleague and seek advice. Each NHS Trust will have a named professional for child protection who can be called upon in such circumstances.

Another group of nurses who may be involved in the early identification of child abuse are school nurses, particularly as a result of their evolving role with individual children in prevention and health promotion. Vizard and Tranter (1988) discuss, in relation to sexual abuse, how children may present at school with academic under-achievement and behavioural disturbances. In the 5–12 year age group they describe how physical signs such as recurrent abdominal pain, bedwetting and soiling, as well as over sexualized behaviour which encroaches into drawings and play, can be indicative of abuse. The 12–18 year group are far more likely to tell someone about their experiences. Vizard and Tranter warn that these adolescents may only attempt to make a disclosure once or maybe twice and they may then give up. It is important, therefore that children are believed. Vizard and Tranter also identify, in this age group, that there appear to be links between sexual abuse, anorexia nervosa and self-mutilating behaviours.

School nurses may be alerted to the possibility of child abuse, particularly sexual abuse, by teachers who are the only professionals who are in regular contact with school age children (Peake, 1995). It is important that school nurses respond promptly when teachers raise concerns about individual children, and they should, if necessary, consult with the NHS community trust's child protection advisor. In some cases, schools will have developed a whole-school policy for dealing with child protection issues in conjunction with social services (Peake, 1995). Where such policies exist, school nurses should ensure that they are familiar with them and abide by them, but that they do not breach their own employer's policies in doing so. It is worth ensuring that the NHS community trust's child protection advisor knows of school policies where they exist so that school nurses are clear as to what actions they should take when concerns are raised.

Pre-school children, who may come to the attention of the health visitor via vigilant nursery teachers or childminders, may also present with unusual behaviour. Vizard and Tranter (1988) describe how this group may present with symptoms such as compulsive masturbation, venereal infections and unusual behaviour. Unusual parent–child interactions may also be noticed. Vizard and Tranter emphasize the importance of realizing that signs in a child may be indicative of problems. A single sign or a transient behaviour change should not be taken as proof of abuse but should make nurses vigilant. If they have any doubts they should discuss their suspicions with a senior manager.

PREDICTIVE FACTORS

Another way of dealing with the problem of child abuse is to try and predict it in advance by identifying those families who may be at risk. To this end a number of factors have been identified which have been shown to be related to abuse. The health visitor's role, in collecting information relating to these factors, is crucial, even if some of it is impressionistic. It is important, however, to see the task of prevention as multidisciplinary, involving social, health and educational professionals. This makes it imperative that nurses understand not only their own role but those of other professionals involved and according to Hallett (1995) most professionals involved in child protection (the exception being general practitioners) are indeed very clear about mutual roles.

A fascinating aspect of Dingwall's (1983b) study was the description of how health visitors interpreted social information in evaluating families that were potentially at risk. Apparently the decision-making process was affected by two factors; the materialistic aspect of the environment and the interpersonal behaviour of the parents. Hence, on the one hand they tended to evaluate whether the home was clean, the state of the children's clothes and if the family were using money wisely, especially if resources were limited. On the other hand, they reacted to such factors as, for example, whether there was a history of drunkenness or crime. Despite this, it was also found that health visitors tended to view parents as respectable and morally responsible unless shown otherwise, and therefore sought justification for any discrepancies in their provision or behaviour from the cultural norms of the environment.

The mother–child bond discussed in Chapter 2 was felt to be of considerable importance by the health visitors involved in the study, perhaps overriding a more objective evaluation of the situation. Kempe and Kempe (1978) in their seminal work on child abuse suggested that there are a number of factors which increase the likelihood of abuse. They point out that none of the problems which arise are of a very practical nature, and include the mother being ill during pregnancy, a prolonged and difficult birth, congenital malformations, birth injuries and prematurity. Also listed are a number of factors in the parents' history which are predictive. These include psychological disturbance, being abused themselves whilst children, being under severe stress and experiencing difficulty in forming a relationship with the child. Since the publication of Kempe and Kempe's work further research has been undertaken which has attempted to refine predictive factors. In a review of this research Browne (1995) concludes that there are five aspects which should be considered when assessing the safety of a child:

1. Knowledge and attitudes towards child rearing – abusing parents tend to have 'unrealistic and distorted' expectations of their

children which influences their views on discipline and punishment. Such families are likely to view child rearing as a simple task and lack awareness of their children's needs.

2. Parental perceptions of child behaviour – abusing parents tend to view their children as more irritable and demanding than non-abusing parents. They may view normal behaviour as being deliberately non-compliant to their wishes.

3. Parental emotions and responses to stress – abusive parents tend to show poorer response to stress and are more likely to be harsher with their children, choosing less appropriate methods of disciplining their children. When children do not respond to demands the parents become increasingly stressed and are more likely to try to resolve the situation with violence. Furthermore, abusing parents tend to be less consistent in terms of discipline, and may respond severely to relatively minor behaviour problems in the child, but allow more serious behaviour problems to go unattended.

4. Parent–child interaction and behaviour – abusive parents tend to show less interactive behaviours with their children and are more likely to be negative and controlling.

5. Quality of child and parent attachment – there is considerable evidence to suggest that there is a link between abuse as a child and abusing behaviour as an adult, which is the result of a failure to form a secure attachment.

Further research in this area (Thoburn *et al.*, 1995) identifies further factors including unemployment, mental health problems in the parents (including substance abuse and immaturity of personality), parental learning disability and a serious loss by the parents (through death or divorce) or serious accident or illness.

There are checklists, which include similar predictive factors to those mentioned above, which can be (and are) used by health care professionals to assess the vulnerability of children. These can serve as a useful indicator for community nurses to the kind of factors which need some consideration. The suggestion that it is possible to use predictive factors lists for the purpose of screening families and identifying potential abusers has, however, been received with much scepticism. Dubowitz (1990) emphasizes that, while abusers may have many common attributes, clinicians believe that 'multiple and interacting factors are usually involved'. He writes (p. 992):

> For example, although the stresses of poverty appear to contribute substantially to child maltreatment, and it might be argued constitute societal maltreatment per se the relationship between poverty and maltreatment is not linear; many poor people are excellent parents.

Browne (1989) also discusses screening using predictive lists. In his study, he involved health visitors in a retrospective evaluation, using a compilation checklist, and compared factors present in known abusing families with non-abusing families. While the predictive list was shown to be a sensitive screening tool, with 82 per cent of abusing families identified and 88 per cent of non-abusing families identified, Browne discusses the problem of 'missing' 18 per cent of abusing families and of falsely identifying 12 per cent of non-abusing families as potential abusers. He suggests the use of a 'second screen' to be undertaken 3–6 months after birth on all those identified as being 'at risk'. This second screen should distinguish between the actual positives and the false positives. A third stage at approximately 9–12 months would assess the child's attachment to the mother or primary caregiver. Underlying this kind of approach is the philosophy that all children are at risk unless there is evidence to the contrary, a view to which some nurses may not wish to subscribe.

Barker (1990) goes as far as to warn against adopting such a philosophy. He discusses Browne's research and emphasizes that:

> ...*there are grave ethical and practical doubts about any behavioural labelling process which enables professionals to point to hitherto blameless families as potential abusers.*

Barker suggests that a more effective strategy would be to offer 'caring support, information and encouragement' to families living in areas of social deprivation. The professional judgement of health visitors, their extensive training and their experience should be utilized in identifying families at risk. Only if health visitors had clear information relating to actual and potential abuse would 'labelling' occur. Clearly there is much debate and controversy about the use of vulnerability checklists and we would suggest that if used in a sensible and sensitive way they can be useful in identifying families who may require additional support. They should not be used without consideration of the context in which assessment is taking place nor should professionals ignore the changes which take place within families which might affect, positively or negatively, their ability in terms of functioning or dysfunctioning. With or without checklists, at all levels, nursing personnel have a considerable role to play in predicting child abuse and nurse educators should teach to this end.

INTERVENTION

The area of intervention is one in which there has been less active involvement from nurses. Similarly, there have been fewer studies investigating their potential involvement. Hopefully, once their role in helping to identify and prevent child abuse becomes more established, we will witness an increased involvement in this important area. However careful we are in trying to prevent abuse, it is unfortunately still likely to occur.

The key to nurses taking a more active role in child abuse stems from training. The lessons of Cleveland outlined in the Butler-Sloss report (1988) show that if professionals are to be involved in such a sensitive field they must have adequate training. Area Child Protection Committees (ACPCs) which exist in all local authorities, and which include representatives from both medicine and nursing, social services, education and the police have a responsibility for 'scrutinising the work related to interagency training' (Dimond, 1996). Most ACPCs have a training sub-committee which will organize and oversee local multidisciplinary training initiatives, which are seen as key to the successful operation of the child protection system (Hallett, 1995; DoH/Welsh Office, 1995).

One aspect of the nursing role which might be further developed is that of educating parents for parenthood. Frude emphasized the importance of this for future generations in 1980 and the community nurse was and still is well placed to take on this role. The nurse may be the first and most regular contact person for the 'at risk' family and has a potentially valuable role to play. In particular it is suggested that the nurse has a strong educative function to play in providing knowledge of child development; in helping with child management training by placing special emphasis on positive interactions; and by implementing self-control training for abusive parents. These components, it is thought, can be successfully combined into a single training programme for abusive parents. This approach extends the traditional role of the community nurse.

A further extension of this role would be to become more involved in the education of children. Community nurses can work with teachers to develop education programmes about sexual abuse, which are appropriate for the age and culture of the children. Wynne (in Potrykus, 1989) suggests that children should be made aware that their bodies are their own. Even from the age of 7 or 8 they need to have knowledge about their bodies. By the time they reach adolescence, education can be more comprehensive but the message is the same.

Nurses also have an important role in the treatment of families where abuse has occurred. Wynne (in Potrykus, 1989) believes that in cases of sexual abuse the health visitor has an important role in helping the mother establish family relationships again. Mothers may feel extreme guilt and disbelief if they have not been aware that abuse was going on, a point which is vividly demonstrated in research by Farmer and Owen (1995). The Butler-Sloss report (1988) also found that in some cases mothers were totally unaware of problems. One woman was married to a man convicted of child sexual abuse and did not know about his past criminal record. These families will need extensive help, and health visitors should liaise with the child psychiatry team about appropriate interventions. Nicol (1989) discusses the many difficulties faced by families and outlines the potential involvement of the child psychiatrist. The health visitor should complement work by other health professionals which will mean constant communication.

Whatever role health visitors, community nurses and hospital based nurses have in the intervention of child abuse, they will be involved in working as part of a team with the family. As members of the multidisciplinary team, nurses should remember the conclusions of the Butler-Sloss report (1988) which emphasized that members should have a clear understanding of each other's role and should communicate with other agencies and within disciplines. Nurses clearly have a role with intervention in child abuse and maybe, in the future, they will become more involved and establish themselves as indispensable members of the multidisciplinary team.

In practice ➤	

- Nurses should exercise extreme caution in making judgements about other people and in predicting their behaviour. Although checklists are useful in alerting nurses to those children potentially at risk, too much reliance must not be placed on them.
- At all times nursing staff need to ensure that the physical and psychological care of the child is put first in any decisions they may make concerning potential abuse in the family.
- Consideration should be given to making greater links between hospital and community staff, especially concerning the admittance and regular appearance of children in accident and emergency departments.
- In dealing with child abuse a multidisciplinary approach is necessary. Consequently, nurses need to be informed and in empathy with the role of other professions, especially social workers and psychologists.
- Nurses might consider extending their role in working with families where child abuse has occurred to include treatment and management. Community nurses especially are very well placed to fulfil this function.
- Nurses should be trained for and encouraged to take a more active educational role in their work with parents. This should be seen as one of the areas of expertise of nurses who specialize in working with children.

REFERENCES

Barker, W. (1990) Practical and ethical doubts about screening for child abuse. *Health Visitor*, **63**(1), 14–17.

Browne, K. (1989) The health visitor's role in screening for child abuse. *Health Visitor*, **62**(9), 275–7.

Browne, K. (1995) Child abuse: Defining, Understanding and Intervening, in *The Child Protection Handbook*, (eds K. Wilson and A. James), Baillière Tindall, London.

Butler-Sloss, E. (1988) *Report of the Inquiry into Child Abuse in Cleveland, 1987*, HMSO, London.

Clothier, C., Macdonald, C.A. and Shaw, D.A. (1994) *The Allitt Inquiry: Independent Inquiry relating to deaths and injuries on the children's ward at*

Grantham and Kesteven General Hospital during the period February to April 1991, HMSO, London.

Corby, B. (1995) Interprofessional Co-operation and Interagency Co-ordination, in *The Child Protection Handbook*, (eds K. Wilson and A. James), Baillière Tindall, London.

Department of Health (1989) *The Children Act*, HMSO, London.

Department of Health and The Welsh Office (1995) *Child Protection: Clarification of Arrangements between the NHS and other Agencies*, HMSO, London.

Dimond, B. (1996) *The Legal Aspects of Child Health Care*, Mosby, London.

Dingwall, R. (1983a) 1. Detecting child abuse. *Nursing Times*, 79(24), 66, 68–9.

Dingwall, R. (1983b) 2. Child abuse: the real questions. *Nursing Times* 79(25), 67–8.

Dubowitz, H. (1990) Pediatrician's role in preventing child maltreatment. *Pediatric Clinics of North America*, 37(4), 989–1002.

Farmer, E. and Owen, M. (1995) *Child Protection Practice: Private Risks and Public Remedies*, Studies in Child Protection Series, HMSO, London.

Frude, N. (1980) A psychological perspective on child abuse, in *Psychological Approaches to Child Abuse*, (ed. N. Frude), Batsford, London.

Ghate, D. and Spencer, L. (1995) *The Prevalence of Child Sexual Abuse in Britain*, HMSO, London.

Gibbons, J., Gallagher, B., Bell, C. and Gordon, D. (1995a) *Development After Physical Abuse in Early Childhood*, Studies in Child Protection Series, HMSO, London.

Gibbons, J., Conroy, S. and Bell, C. (1995b) *Operating the Child Protection System*, Studies in Child Protection Series, HMSO, London.

Hallett, C. (1995) *Interagency Coordination in Child Protection*, Studies in Child Protection Series, HMSO, London.

Hobbs, C. J. and Wynne, J.M. (1990) The sexually abused battered child. *Archives of Disease in Childhood*, 65, 423–7.

Home Office, Department of Health, Department of Education and Science and The Welsh Office (1991) *Working Together Under the Children Act: A Guide to Arrangements for Interagency Co-operation for the Protection of Children from Abuse*, HMSO, London.

Jackson, C. (1989) Pack up your troubles. *Health Visitor*, 62(9), 264.

Kempe, R.S. and Kempe, C.H. (1978) *Child Abuse*, Fontana/Open Books, London.

Kent, A. (1988) Health visitors or child police? *Nursing Times*, 84(1), 18.

Meadow, R. (1989) Munchausen's syndrome by proxy, in *ABC of Child Abuse*, (ed. R. Meadow), British Medical Journal, London.

Millor, G.K. (1981) A theoretical framework for nursing research in child abuse and neglect. *Nursing Research*, 30(2), 78–83.

Nicol, A.R. (1989) Role of the child psychiatry team, in *ABC of Child Abuse*, (ed. R. Meadow), British Medical Journal, London.

Parker, R. (1995) A brief history of Child Protection, in *1995 Child Protection Practice: Private Risks and Public Remedies*, (E. Farmer and M. Owen), Studies in Child Protection Series, HMSO, London.

Peake, A. (1995) Dealing with suspicion of child sexual abuse: the role of the teacher, in *The Child Protection Handbook*, (eds K. Wilson and A. James), Baillière Tindall, London.

Potrykus, C. (1989) Piecing together the jigsaw of child protection. *Health Visitor*, 62(9), 278–9.

Sharman, R.L. (1983) *Child Abuse: a Discussion Paper* Council for the Education and Training of Health Visitors, London.

Stockell, F. (1972) *The Unpopular Patient*, RCN, London.

Taylor, S. and Tilley, N. (1989) Health visitors and child protection: conflict, contradictions and ethical dilemmas. *Health Visitor*, 62(9), 273–5.

Thoburn, J., Lewis, A. and Shemmings, D. (1995) *Paternalism or Partnership? Family Involvement in the Child Protection Process*, Studies in Child Protection Series, HMSO, London.

Vizard, E. and Tranter, M. (1988) Recognition and assessment of child sexual abuse, in *Child Sexual Abuse Within the Family: Assessment and Treatment*, (eds A. Bentovim, A. Elton, J. Hildebrand, M. Tranter and E. Vizard), John Wright, London.

Wattley, L.A. and Müller, D.J. (1984) *Investigating Psychology: A Practical Approach for Nursing*, Harper and Row, London.

FURTHER READING

Frude, N. (1990) *Understanding family problems: a psychological approach*, John Wiley, Chichester.

Kempe, R.S. and Kempe, C.H. (1978) *Child Abuse*, Fontana/Open Books, London.

Although slightly dated still the best short introductory text on child abuse. Very easy to read and full of interest.

Millor, G.K. (1981) A theoretical framework for nursing research in child abuse and neglect. *Nursing Research*, 30, 78–83.

A specialized paper for nurse researchers with interests in the area of child abuse and neglect.

Wilson, K. and James, A. (eds) *The Child Protection Handbook*, Baillière Tindall, London.

This excellent book reviews much of the recent research in the field of child protection including studies which formed part of the Studies in Child Protection Series. It has some unusual contributions including a look at the teacher's role and aspects of working with abused children.

CHILDREN AND ADOLESCENTS WITH HIV INFECTION

14

The importance of a research base which can guide nursing practice has been referred to constantly throughout this book. If the research base does not exist or is in the process of being developed there will inevitably be confusion about practice.

Research which looks at the psychological care of children with human immunodeficiency virus (HIV) has been far from plentiful. The early association of HIV infection with homosexuality, promiscuity and drug abuse resulted in many nurses involved in child care feeling remote from the epidemic. When it became evident that children were being infected more research was undertaken but it tended to be orientated towards physical care and infection control. As more nurses become involved with HIV infected children, it is hoped that more research looking at their psychological needs will be undertaken. The aim of this chapter is to look at the psychological implications of HIV infection in children and to discuss how nurses can prepare themselves for their roles as both carers and educators. The emphasis throughout is on family care because most children acquire the virus from their seropositive mothers *in utero* and at birth. HIV is one of only a few life threatening diseases that potentially can affect all members of a family. Many infected children and their mothers, as well as fathers and siblings who are seropositive, will eventually develop acquired immunodeficiency syndrome (AIDS) and many will die. Nurses who are involved in the care of children with AIDS will not be able to ignore the needs of other members of the family who may also be sick. The provision of total family care will challenge many existing health care services and nurses must be prepared for radical changes in practice.

CHILDREN AT RISK

Children become infected with HIV in the following ways:

1. by acquiring the virus from their infected mothers during pregnancy, at birth, or, rarely, through breast milk (perinatal transmission);
2. through receipt of infected blood, blood products, bone marrow and organs;
3. through sharing needles with infected drug users; and
4. through sexual contact with an infected person.

Perinatal infection from HIV infected mothers

In 1983 scientists at the Centers for Communicable Diseases in the United States identified that some children born to HIV infected mothers were infected with the virus. Stine (1997) reports that currently in the United States over 90 per cent of children with HIV infection became infected by so called 'vertical transmission' – that is infection through their mothers either *in utero*, at birth or rarely through breast milk.

In the United Kingdom, the numbers of HIV positive women are steadily rising. The consequence of this increase will mean that the largest proportion of children with HIV infection will, in future, become infected during the perinatal period.

Studies worldwide have shown that there is wide geographic variation in transmission rates from HIV infected mothers to their babies with rates varying from between 15 per cent in Europe to 59 per cent in Africa (Stine, 1997). Many of these women engage in 'high risk' behaviour, that is sexual contact with intravenous drug users, being users themselves, or both. Many of these women only become aware that they are infected when their child becomes ill and is diagnosed as being HIV infected. These mothers not only have to adjust to the knowledge that they are infected, but that they have also passed the virus on to their child. Nunes *et al.* (1995) describe the intense feelings, devastation and acute responses of people when they are told of their diagnosis. Reactions at the time include anger, anxiety and fear because of the potentially poor prognosis and 'questionable future'.

Handyside (1995) emphasizes the importance of counselling at the time of diagnosis as service users' first impressions can 'influence their decisions about later (service) use' (p. 209).

Nurses involved with families at the time of diagnosis should be aware of how families may react when they are told the 'bad news' and during the period of adaptation which will inevitably be traumatic. Miller (1988) suggests that as patients adjust to the diagnosis they tend to try and hide their personal distress in order to try and protect their children. This can result in greater 'emotional, psychological, psychiatric and even physical distress'. Miller feels that patients will need time to discuss their anxieties and will need to have their diagnosis put into perspective (see Miller, 1987, 1988 for further discussion). Hayter (1994) discusses other feelings felt by parents such as guilt, anger, fear and sometimes blame (e.g. who infected who). Families who have a child infected through hospital controlled blood or blood products may also feel extreme anger towards health care workers.

Blood and blood products

The first description of AIDS in a child was in 1982 (Prose, 1990). The child, from San Francisco USA, was thought to have acquired the infection after receiving a blood transfusion. By 1983 children with haemophilia had become infected with HIV in alarming proportions after receiving contaminated Factor VIII, a vital clotting component of blood. It became evident in the USA and the UK that the supply of blood for transfusion and for the manufacture of blood products was heavily contaminated with the virus. The sad irony was that the availability of

Factor VIII a decade before had promised to help children and adults with haemophilia lead relatively unrestricted lifestyles.

Since 1986 in Britain (and since 1985 in the USA) all blood has been tested for the presence of antibodies and Factor VIII is treated to inactivate viruses. These measures have substantially reduced the risk of contracting HIV through blood. These processes are, however, expensive and are not being carried out worldwide. Stine (1997) reports that in many developing countries blood and blood products still account for between 5 and 10 per cent of HIV infection.

Donated organs and bone marrow are also a potential source of infection in children, although the risk is minimal. Since this mode of transmission was recognized, organs and bone marrow are tested for antibodies, although a small risk remains (Stine, 1997). Nurses may, however, come into contact with children infected in this way.

Intravenous drug users

While the future is brighter for children in the developed world born with haemophilia and those who may require blood transfusions, there is still a group of children and adolescents for whom the risk of becoming infected has not lessened. These are the intravenous drug users who account, for example, for 17 per cent of HIV infections among teenagers in the USA. Peer conformity is often described as a factor of adolescence (Taylor and Muller, 1995), with the adolescent conforming to the values of the peer group, and it has been suggested as a reason why young people may take drugs. Risk behaviour (such as drug use) is also seen as a 'key feature' of adolescence (Bagnall and Dilloway, 1997). Mussen *et al.* (1990), in their review of research about the personality of drug abusers, identify that they are usually impulsive, disorganized in thinking, superficial and sporadic in their relationships. Oppenheimer's (1985) review of British studies which looked at personality of adolescent drug users found that they tend to score above the norm for neuroticism, and score below the norm for 'obedience'.

While the dark world of drug dealing may seem very remote from the average children's ward or child care unit, some of these young people will eventually arrive in hospital where they will present a great challenge for all health care workers and their carers. There is clearly a role here too in terms of health promotion, particularly for school nurses and health visitors. Bagnall and Dilloway (1997) emphasize that drug use in schools is a reality but stress that further research into misuse is required because it occurs due to a host of 'individual and complex issues' (p. 22). One important service which is having a potential effect in terms of reducing infections, and of which adolescents need to be made aware, if they are using drugs, is the needle exchange programme which has become widespread throughout the UK. Unfortunately, however, as is generally the case, those at greatest risk are those who are least likely to participate in such schemes (Stine, 1997).

Infection through sexual contact

Sexual abuse of children is discussed in Chapter 13. There is limited evidence that children have become infected with HIV through sexual abuse (Stine, 1997), although sexual abuse is clearly a potential mode of transmission. However, as the virus becomes more widespread throughout the heterosexual population, the risk to children who are abused sexually will undoubtedly become greater.

It is not only children who are sexually abused who are at risk of contracting HIV infection. The sexual habits of adolescents have been subject to much speculation, although few reliable studies have been carried out largely because this is a difficult area to investigate (Dockrell and Joffe, 1992). However, Stine (1997) cites evidence from the USA showing that over half the teenagers aged between 13 and 19 years have had sex by the age of 16 years and 70 per cent are sexually active by the age of 19 years. These young people are putting themselves at risk and recent data show that 60 per cent of new HIV infections globally occur among young women aged between 15 and 24 years (Stine, 1997). Furthermore, in the USA a quarter of new infections are thought to occur in those between 13 and 20 years. There is an obvious need for AIDS education in schools if this mode of transmission in young people is to be contained. Such education should form part of the wider agenda of sex education although such programmes are not without their problems (Taylor and Müller, 1995; Cohen, 1994; O'Driscoll, 1997). A number of innovative schemes for providing such education are running in the UK and elsewhere and we await with interest data from these programmes (Carlisle, 1997; ICN, 1997; Payne, 1994; O'Driscoll, 1997).

It should not be assumed that all adolescent sexual contact is always part of the experimentation which occurs as the adolescent searches for identity. Moriasy and Thomas (1990) report that in many cultures it is not unusual for young people to marry and have children of their own in their early adolescence. While cultural constraints determine that girls should be virgins upon marriage, the same is often not true for boys who are expected to be sexually experienced when they enter marriage. Whatever the reason for young adolescents becoming sexually active, the risks are great. Moriasy and Thomas (1990) write (p. 21):

> *Clearly, throughout the world, whatever the prevailing social norm, many young unmarried people do engage in sexual activity, some at very young ages and many with a high degree of ignorance about how to avoid unwanted pregnancy or sexually transmitted diseases, including HIV infection.*

HIV INFECTION AND CHILD DEVELOPMENT

As more children became infected with HIV, scientists realized that the retrovirus behaves differently in children. The Centers for Disease

Control have acknowledged these differences, and in 1987 developed a classification system for children with HIV infection (see Hayter, 1994). It has also been identified that the time between becoming infected with the virus and developing AIDS is considerably less in children than in adults. Prose (1990) states that the majority of children infected perinatally will develop symptoms of AIDS infection within two years of birth. Hayter cites evidence suggesting that of children infected perinatally 25 per cent will develop AIDS in the first year of life, and a further 15 per cent by the end of second year of life. In subsequent years the rate of progression to AIDS is about 10 per cent. Symptoms vary considerably from child to child and the effects on development very much depend on how the disease presents. The earliest sign of AIDS in infancy is pneumocystis carinii (Stine, 1997; Kelnar *et al.*, 1995) which is the most common opportunistic infection found in children with AIDS. Prose (1990) reports that the majority of children with AIDS in the USA have central nervous system involvement and show signs of progressive neurological dysfunction including developmental delay. Children with AIDS also experience failure to thrive, lymphoid interstitial pneumonia and/or pulmonary lymphoid hyperplasia, bacterial and opportunistic infections and secondary cancers.

The range of potential symptoms make the disease course almost impossible to predict which causes added trauma for the family. Hayter (1994) suggests that parents of affected children found that not knowing about their child's condition was extremely stressful. The unpredictable nature of HIV infection makes it very difficult for parents to have any certain knowledge of the future. With older children who are HIV infected, parents find it difficult to answer their child's questions honestly and this can affect the child–parent relationship.

Where symptoms such as failure to thrive do present in younger children, it is difficult to distinguish between symptomatic HIV infection and other childhood illness which is not attributed to HIV infection. Parents, as well as nurses and health visitors, must not make assumptions that all ailments are HIV related. Becoming over protective each time a child shows signs of minor illness can positively reinforce illness behaviour, and a child may learn that such behaviour is rewarded with attention and therefore repeat it. Overreaction to minor illness by parents can also distort the child's understanding of the 'sick role'. Parmelee (1989) describes how parental reactions to minor illness can influence the way children cope 'emotionally and cognitively' with more severe illness. Health visitors and nurses must be aware of the need for parents to behave in an appropriate way to minor illness although this may be very difficult for parents as even minor symptoms can provoke intense anxiety (Hayter, 1994). The provision of support and direction is vital to the successful outcome of a period of illness. Many children will eventually develop AIDS and it will be important for both the child and the parents to have a relationship which will be able to withstand the stresses of more severe and potentially life threatening episodes.

When children are HIV infected and have remained asymptomatic, parents may be reluctant to allow their child to join in with childhood activities in case they inadvertently become exposed to illness. It is important, however, that children who are HIV infected do not become socially isolated because of parental fears and anxieties. Peer group interaction and its influences on social and emotional development cannot be overestimated (see Chapter 3). Children should have the opportunity to mix with other children, which will involve attending schools, playgroups and nurseries. Exclusions from school should be as few as possible because if older children do not attend school they can potentially underachieve academically, lose friends and peer support and become even more socially isolated. Leiderman (1989) identifies even toddlers and pre-school children as needing peer affiliation. If they do not interact with peers and near peers they may exhibit inappropriate behaviour and be deficient in relationship skills.

TO TEST OR NOT

The decision to test a child to find out if he or she is HIV infected is a difficult one to make. Many parents feel they would rather not know because if the result is positive they will be constantly watching for signs that their child has developed AIDS. A positive diagnosis in a child will also confirm the mother's positive status (Hayter, 1994). Mothers who are aware that they are HIV infected should be told that serological testing of babies until they have reached 18 months old to two years is, in any case, inexact. The conventional HIV test is not reliable because babies born to HIV infected mothers have maternal anti-HIV IgG transmitted passively through the placenta (Stine, 1997). Many of these babies will not develop their own anti-HIV antibodies and any test done in the presence of maternal anti-HIV IgG will show as a false positive result in the baby. Maternal anti-HIV IgG may persist until the baby is two years old (Stine, 1997) and many mothers have been faced with having to wait to discover whether their babies have anti-HIV antibodies themselves and are therefore HIV infected. Work is currently under way to find accurate ways of confirming the diagnosis. This is important because of the need to commence prophylactic treatment in babies who are definitely HIV positive, while at the same time avoiding unnecessary and potentially toxic therapy in children who are definitely negative. The psychological trauma of having to wait for so long has been severe for infected mothers but the risk of false results has made the wait very necessary.

Parents who do take the decision to have their children tested will require skilled counselling prior to the test and when they receive the results. If test results are positive, the family should be helped to make decisions about appropriate medical interventions. Elliott (1987) emphasizes that it is important for nurses to recognize their professional limitations and they should, with the permission of the family, seek specialist help if required. The role of the clinical psychologist is discussed fully by Miller (1987), and Miller and Brown (1988). There are also many organizations offering a range of counselling and support services that parents may wish to contact.

Even if test results are negative, parents who are positive themselves will need to discuss the implications for themselves and the child. Follow up testing of children at regular intervals is usually carried out to monitor the health status of the child. Each time the child is tested, the family will be subjected to fear and anxiety. Nurses and health visitors may well be involved with the family during these stressful times, and it is vital that there is careful liaison between all professional and voluntary groups with the family. Clinics should operate 'open door' policies so that families can seek support at any time (Hayter, 1994).

WHO NEEDS TO KNOW?

Jones (1990) who has worked extensively with children and adults with haemophilia in the North of England discusses the difficulties faced by parents who have to tell a child that they are HIV infected. He has found that children often know more than their parents think they know and while the telling is traumatic, once the truth has been shared the whole family can benefit. He writes (p. 197):

> One youngster said that he had not wanted to frighten his parents by telling them that he knew. Another said he thought that nobody had dared to tell him because all the news was bad and he was going to die soon.

There is also a risk that the child could learn about his or her HIV status from a third person which could be potentially very damaging (Hayter, 1994). This may seem unlikely in view of professional confidentiality and yet Green and Platt (1997) reported some very worrying data indicating that among the respondents they interviewed who were HIV positive, one fifth reported breaches of confidentiality.

Apart from the children themselves it is difficult to know who else to tell. Children and families may be stigmatized and isolated because of the ignorance and fear of others. Logan et al. (1990) described the discrimination suffered by some children with haemophilia when:

> ...public panic and outrage did not distinguish children with haemophilia from other groups at high risk of HIV infection.

This panic was widespread with reports of other parents keeping their children away from school rather than let them come into contact with an HIV infected child. Gulland (1997) found that children preferred to tell others that they had cancer or a blood disorder rather than HIV because of their fear of becoming outcasts. The effects of this stigma on children has not been studied on a wide scale although Logan et al. (1990) studied the psychological morbidity among a group of school-aged boys with haemophilia in Scotland. Their findings did not show any significant problems.

Parents of infected children have to consider carefully the implications of telling the staff of schools, nurseries and playgroups. It is well documented that transmission does not occur during normal social contact and in any case universal precautions such as careful handwashing should be adopted when dealing with body fluids. Certainly many consider that it is not necessary for teaching staff at school to know and it is not a legal requirement that teachers are told (Jones, 1990). However, parents must consider that it could be of value to a child if a caring and sensitive teacher did know. Thurtle (1997), in a discussion of the teacher's role with ill children, emphasizes the importance of their influence within the school setting. A teacher who is aware of the diagnosis can do a great deal to minimize the emotional trauma for children who are aware that they are HIV infected. For example, a child may become distressed by AIDS-related issues discussed formally in class or informally among peers. A teacher could be very supportive at times such as this. Teachers who are told the diagnosis of a child may need practical advice from the school nurse about how to cope in first aid situations as well as help in coming to terms with personal fears and prejudices.

THE IMPLICATIONS FOR NURSES

By its very nature HIV infection and AIDS will more and more involve whole families. Pizzo (1990) in the United States and Mok (1988) in Scotland identify that a diagnosis of HIV infection in a child usually means that the family is also infected. In the two decades since the first identification of AIDS it has become clear that existing hospital and community services need to adapt radically in order to meet the needs of families with more than one infected symptomatic member. In Chapter 12 the family consequences of caring for a child with chronic illness are described. If adults, as well as children from the same family have to, for example, attend different clinics and hospital departments, and see different doctors, the consequences are much worse. Wards and departments need to offer services for families with HIV infection as a whole rather than for individuals. What is also apparent is that families need community based services which can offer more flexible and accessible services (Handyside, 1995). Nurses who work with families in the community, such as health visitors, community child care nurses and school nurses, have found that their role has had to change radically. They have had to take on a more generic role and look at the needs of the family unit rather than at individuals. Such families put strain on already stretched community health and social services. Families need practical help as well as counselling and emotional support which requires special nursing skills. If nurses take on this supportive role, it is important that they possess the necessary skills so that they are effective. These skills involve counselling and an ability to know when families need specialist help from, for example, a clinical psychologist. It is also vitally important that they keep up to date with information about HIV and AIDS. Key workers play an important role with families to ensure that families are empowered and are able to remain the principal decision-makers in terms of their own care (Hayter, 1994).

When talking to families, hospital and community nurses must be careful not to be judgemental about the lifestyles and habits of those in their care. All nurses need to examine their own feelings about the virus and resolve their fears and prejudices before they are confronted with a situation that could potentially be very damaging to a family who have already suffered discrimination from others. As Hayter (1994) writes 'AIDS awareness is very often self-awareness' (p. 220). Kennedy and Chester (1997) recognize the stress on health care professionals who are involved in the care of patients with HIV and AIDS and recommend that staff support systems should be established in order to prevent staff distress. They describe such a system operating among a group of HIV maternity counsellors in London who, like many community based practitioners, can find themselves isolated through the very nature of their work. Education is key in meeting the needs of families and should focus upon self-care and the care and support of colleagues as well as upon the psychosocial needs of families (Nunes *et al.*, 1995).

Fostering and adoption

Inevitably, in families with more than one infected person, deaths may occur leaving a bereaved parent or an orphaned child. The children who survive their parents will need special care. Fostering and adoption programmes are being pioneered in the USA where an estimated 24 600 children and 21 000 adolescents had been orphaned by the HIV/AIDS epidemic by the end of 1995 (Stine, 1997). Such programmes are vital as a way of preventing large numbers of children living, and possibly dying, in residential care.

The effects of institutional living are discussed by Hersov (1985) who cites studies which have found that children in residential care have significantly higher incidences of emotional and behavioural problems. Fostering programmes should prevent the adverse effects of institutional care on child development. However, Hersov discusses studies which have identified the high failure rate of foster placements (one study found a 48 per cent failure rate). Clearly potential foster parents need skilled counselling prior to taking on the care of a child with HIV infection. It is known that many children who are infected with HIV will go on to develop AIDS although the uncertain incubation period makes it difficult to make accurate predictions. AIDS manifests itself in many ways and these children need a great deal of physical and psychological care. If they develop AIDS they will almost inevitably die (Stine, 1997). Health visitors, school nurses and community child care nurses can provide practical and psychological support for both foster parents and children.

A DUTY TO CARE

The challenge of responding to the care of families with HIV and AIDS is mounting (Nunes *et al.*, 1995). Nurses who are faced with caring for an HIV infected child and family for the first time may initially feel apprehensive about their role. AIDS and HIV have attracted a massive amount of media attention, most of which has linked HIV to homosexuality, drug abuse and promiscuity. Such negative media images have led to concern and to overzealous infection control measures. Green and Platt (1997) found, in their study of the views of HIV positive respondents about health care workers, that many had experienced incidents where health care workers had tried to avoid contact with them either by refusing to treat them adequately or by wearing protecting clothing or by physically isolating them. The UKCC (1992) has, however, condemned such practices and sets out clear guidelines regarding the care of HIV positive people.

HIV infected children who require care have a right to receive that care. Nurses must not condemn them because their mothers are HIV infected or because they have haemophilia and contracted the virus through receiving contaminated blood products. Neither should nurses condemn the family for the values they hold. In 1987 and again in 1992 the United Kingdom Central Council (UKCC) for Nurses, Midwives and Health Visitors issued a statement about the nurse's role in caring for patients with HIV and AIDS (UKCC, 1988; UKCC, 1992; see also Dimond, 1996) which categorically states that nurses cannot be allowed to choose or select which patients they wish to nurse. In 1990 the UKCC Professional Conduct Committee heard its first case of a nurse refusing to care for patients with HIV and AIDS (*Nursing Times* 1990). The nurse was struck off the UKCC register.

'Care', however, is an extremely subjective word – a more suitable term might be that patients have a right to receive 'competent care'. Munley Gallagher (1990) found in her study of health care workers that even after specific education about the transmission of HIV, irrational fears were still prevalent. If fears exist it must be debatable whether nurses can deliver competent care without the child and family being aware of the nurse's anxieties. Nor is it sufficient to meet only the physical needs of patients. Negative attitudes by nursing staff can cause great distress. Nurses need to be aware of, and competent at dealing with, psychological and social needs as well as physical needs (Nunes *et al.*, 1995).

Wells (1988) described the 'Ostrich syndrome', with many health care professionals who have not been involved with patients who are HIV infected refusing to believe that AIDS will ever be a problem to them. However, with a growing incidence of infection among the heterosexual population and the vertical transmission from infected mothers to their children all nurses and health visitors involved in child care must be prepared to meet the challenge of caring for children with HIV and AIDS. Wells defined what this challenge means to nursing in practical terms:

1. meaningful acute care in the hospital and community setting;
2. continuing care;
3. leaving or returning control to the patient;
4. support of those close to the patient;
5. confidentiality; and
6. patient advocacy.

THE NURSE, HIV INFECTION AND HEALTH EDUCATION

All nurses have a role to play in society as health educators – for some (such as health visitors) 'health teaching' is fundamental to their work while for others it may be a less formal role. Informal education can occur when a nurse demonstrates a lifestyle which supports what other health educationists are saying. Of course, if we acknowledge that this informal teaching and learning occurs, we must accept too that nurses can also teach unhealthy behaviours. Information that is disseminated must be accurate. In order to spread accurate knowledge nurses must be in possession of accurate knowledge and it is important that they keep themselves up to date with contemporary health issues. On a more formal basis school nurses, community child care nurses and health visitors are likely to be involved with families in AIDS education. Some clinical nurse specialists and infection control nurses are also involved. There are several groups of people who will be or should be formally educated so that children learn the truth about what HIV is and how to prevent its transmission. These groups include:

1. children of all ages who do not have HIV infection and their families;
2. children who are HIV infected and their families;
3. teachers; and
4. media figures.

Educating children

The Education Act of 1993 made significant amendments to previous legislation including measures affecting sex education in schools. From September 1994 sex education, including information about HIV and AIDS, became mandatory in all state secondary schools (although parents have the right to withdraw their children from such education except where it is part of the National Curriculum) but remains optional in primary schools. Teaching about HIV and AIDS and sexual behaviour was removed from the National Curriculum science course so that it could be placed within a moral framework. Clearly, the school environment is a place where children spend a great deal of time, and it is influential to a child's psychological and social development. The Health Education Authority states that schools should be 'health promoting communities' and should be able to influence not only what goes on in the classroom, but also the child's family and the community. In relation to HIV/AIDS education and sex education in general Cohen (1994) suggests teachers and health professionals should work together to identify the best ways of meeting the needs of an individual school community.

With older children, peer education is one of the most effective ways of changing behaviour. Nurses may be involved in facilitating this educational process and must ensure that accurate, appropriate information is available. Clift *et al.* (1989) undertook a major research project for the AIDS Education Research Unit at Christ Church College, Canterbury. The project involved collecting data relating to the 'knowledge, beliefs, attitudes and behaviours' of adolescents aged between 14 and 18 years about HIV and AIDS. This project details information which has ultimately been of value to health educators when considering educational input to this group. Education must be appropriate, age-specific and effective in changing behaviour. The study contains much useful information for nurses and other health care workers involved with adolescents and is essential reading for all involved in HIV and AIDS education.

Affolter (1989) emphasizes the need to ensure that teaching material is appropriate to the environment. Working in Northern Ireland with adolescents she found that there was nothing suitable for that environment. Ultimately a writing team was set up and a programme designed, tested and introduced.

Children and their families who are infected

Jones (1990) suggests that families will need to talk about their fears and anxieties. Nurses may be involved with counselling families but should only take on that role if they feel that they are competent to do so. Miller (1987) emphasizes that effective counselling requires:

1. a thorough working knowledge of HIV;
2. a working knowledge of the lifestyles of patient groups;
3. a working knowledge of the 'back-up' services available; and
4. the ability to recognize common psychosocial and clinical complications arising from HIV.

Nurses in the community may also have the opportunity to influence other parents about HIV infection. It is important that nurses carefully assess who they're talking to and aim to 'speak the same language as their intended audience' (Moriasy and Thomas, 1990). Written back-up information must also be relevant and appropriate.

Nurses involved in health education must ensure they are aware of what material is available and should be conversant with it. Keeping up to date is essential and health authorities should ensure that provision is made for nurses to update themselves at regular intervals. Munley Gallagher (1990) emphasizes the importance of carers being competent and writes:

If people with AIDS are to receive adequate health care, educated providers must be available. They must overcome learning barriers about AIDs and curricula for educating providers which address the physical and psychological aspects of AIDS must be implemented.

The role of teachers

School nurses are in an ideal position to provide education and support for teachers and other school staff who may be anxious about HIV and AIDS. Teachers are extremely influential in the lives of children and ultimately in society. Mok (1989, p. 165) writes:

> *It is hoped that an enlightened teaching staff will mean a more tolerant society as school children grow up, with less stigma surrounding HIV infected children.*

Media figures

There are many people in the media spotlight who are very influential in the health education of children – for example, pop stars, royalty and presenters of children's television programmes. It is important that these people, who provide role models for many children, are aware of their responsibilities and are encouraged to spread the message about HIV. There are also television programmes which include health issues in them. For example, Eastenders, a popular 'soap opera', reaches millions of viewers each week, including children. Magazines are also a powerful source of information particularly for adolescents. Magazine coverage has however been criticized because although there is a wealth of information about relationships and sexual issues, according to Payne (1994) their coverage of HIV and AIDS related topics leaves 'much to be desired' (p. 12).

◄ In practice

- Nurses should not make judgements about the lifestyles of other people nor should they condemn them for the values they hold.
- Communication between all health workers involved with the family is vital if high-quality care is to be provided. Consideration should be given to specialist workers extending their role so that care to family members is not duplicated by different health professionals.
- Nurses must ensure that they keep up to date with research about the physical, social and psychological care of HIV infected families. They should be actively involved in educating families and others involved in the care of the family.
- The issue of confidentiality is of great importance. Families have a right to confidentiality. Many AIDS patients have suffered discrimination and their rights have been compromised.
- Nurses must be aware of, and explore, their own fears and prejudices. If they think that their fears may interfere with their ability to care competently for families they should seek advice from an appropriate person so that problems can be discussed without families suffering.

REFERENCES

Affolter, S. (1989) Education on AIDS. *Nursing Standard*, 3(37), 51–3.

Bagnall, P. and Dilloway, M. (1997) *In a different light: school nurses and their role in meeting the needs of school-age children*, The Queens Nursing Institute/Department of Health, London.

Carlisle, D. (1997) Unite and Fight. *Nursing Times*, 93(48), 13.

Clift, S., Stears, D., Legg, S., Memon, A. and Ryan, L. (1989) *The HIV/AIDS Education and Young People Project. Report on Phase One*, HIV/AIDS Education Research Unit, Christ Church College, Canterbury.

Cohen, P. (1994) The role of the school nurse in providing sex education. *Nursing Times*, 90(23), 36–7.

Dimond, B. (1996) *Legal Aspects of Child Health Care*, Mosby, London.

Dockrell, J. and Joffe, H. (1992) Methodological issues involving the study of young people and HIV/AIDS: a social psychological view. *Health Education Research*, 7(4), 509–16.

Elliott, J. (1987) Nursing care. *British Medical Journal*, 295, 104–6.

Green, G. and Platt, S. (1997) Fear and Loathing in Health Care Settings reported by people with HIV. *Sociology of Health and Illness* 19(1), 70–92.

Gulland, A. (1997) Growing Pains. *Nursing Times* 93(48), 12.

Handyside, E. (1995) The needs of people with HIV, their informal carers and service providers, in *Researching User Perspectives on Community Health Care*, (ed. B. Heyman), Chapman and Hall, London.

Hayter, M. (1994) The Child with HIV/AIDS, in *Caring for dying children and their families*, (ed. L. Hill), Chapman and Hall, London.

Hersov, L. (1985) Adoption and fostering, in *Child and Adolescent Psychiatry*, (eds M. Rutter and L. Hersov), Blackwell Scientific Publications, Oxford.

ICN (1997) *Healthy Young People – a brighter tomorrow*, ICN International Nurses Day 1997 paper.

Jones, P. (1990) *Living with Haemophilia*, 3rd edn, Castle House Publications, Tunbridge Wells.

Kelnar, C.J.H., Harvey, D. and Simpson, C. (1995) *The Sick Newborn Baby*, 3rd edn, Chapman and Hall, London.

Kennedy, J. and Chester, T. (1997) Professional Support for HIV and Maternity Services. *Nursing Times*, 93(37), 53–4.

Leiderman, P.H. (1989) Relationship disturbances and development through the life cycle, in *Relationship Disturbances in Early Childhood*, (eds A.J. Sameroff and R.D. Emde), Basic Books, New York.

Logan, F.A., MacClean, A., Howie, C.A., Gibson, B., Hann, I.M. and Parry Jones, W.L. (1990) Psychological disturbance in children with haemophilia. *British Medical Journal*, 301, 1253–7.

Miller, D. (1987) Counselling, in *ABC of AIDS*, (ed. M.W. Adler), British Medical Journal, London.

Miller, D. (1988) HIV and social psychiatry, in AIDS and HIV infection: the wider perspective, (eds A.J. Pinching, R.A. Weiss and D. Miller), *British Medical Bulletin*, 44(1), 131–48.

Miller, D. and Brown, B. (1988) Developing the role of clinical psychology in the context of AIDS. *The Psychologist: Bulletin of the British Psychological Society*, 1, 63–6.

Mok, J.Y.A. (1988) Infants of women seropositive for HIV. *Midwife, Health Visitor and Community Nurse*, 24(11), 458–62.

Mok, J.Y.A. (1989) Paediatric HIV infection, in *Counselling in HIV Infection and AIDS*, (eds J. Green and A. McCreaner), Blackwell Scientific Publications, Oxford.

Moriasy, J. and Thomas, L. (1990) *Triple jeopardy – Women and AIDS*, Panos-Books.

Munley Gallagher, R. (1990) AIDS: the fear of contagion. *Nursing Standard*, 4(19), 30–2.

Mussen, P., Conger, J.J., Kagan, J. and Huston, A.C. (1990) *Child Development and Personality*, 7th edn, Harper & Row, New York.

Nunes, J.A., Raymond, S.J., Kenneally, N.P., D'Meza Leuner, J. and Webster, A. (1995) Social Support, quality of life, immune function and health in persons living with HIV. *Journal of Holistic Nursing* 13(2), 174–98.

Nursing Times News (1990) RGN struck off for refusal to treat AIDS. *Nursing Times*, 86(51), 5.

O'Driscoll, M. (1997) Let's talk about sex. *Nursing Times* 93(49), 34–5.

Oppenheimer, E. (1985) Drug taking, in *Child and Adolescent Psychiatry*, (eds M. Rutter and L. Hersov), Blackwell Scientific Publications, Oxford.

Parmelee, A.H. (1989) The child's physical health and the development of relationships, in *Relationship Disturbances in Early Childhood*, (eds A.J. Sameroff and R.D. Emde), Basic Books, New York.

Payne, D. (1994) Glossing over the risks. *Nursing Times*, 93(40), 12–13.

Pizzo, P.A. (1990) Pediatric AIDS, problems within problems. *The Journal of Infectious Diseases*, 161, 316 –25.

Prose, N. (1990) HIV infection in children. *Journal of the American Academy of Dermatology*, 22, 1223–31.

Stine, G.J. (1997) *AIDS Update 1997*, Prentice Hall, New Jersey.

Taylor, J. and Muller, D. (1995) *Nursing Adolescents: Research and Psychological Perspectives*, Blackwell, Oxford.

Thurtle, V. (1997) Multi-disciplinary Care of Sick Children in the Community, in *Early Childhood Studies: an holistic approach*, (eds J. Taylor and M. Woods), Arnold, London.

UKCC (1988) *AIDS and HIV Infection*, Circular no PC/88/03, UKCC, London.

UKCC (1992) *Acquired Immune Deficiency Syndrome and Human Immuno-deficiency Virus Infection*, revised Position Statement, UKCC, London.

Wells, R. (1988) AIDS – are nurses ready to meet the challenge? *Senior Nurse*, 8(1), 6–7.

Stine, G.J. (1997) *AIDS Update 1997*, Prentice Hall, New Jersey.
This now seemingly annual update is both readable and provides up-to-date information on the global picture in terms of incidence and treatment.

FURTHER READING

15 DEATH AND THE DYING CHILD

Any discussion about the needs of the dying child will quickly touch the emotions of not only the reader but also the writers as well. The sudden death of a child, or caring for a dying child, is a very intense and personal experience which is difficult to contemplate. It is probably true to say that only those with first hand experience can really understand the feelings of people facing this situation. Nevertheless, nurses working with children do have to prepare themselves as best they can to deal with the death of a child. The aim of this chapter is to indicate to nurses with limited experience of the dying child some of the issues they must be prepared for, and to offer some helpful and practical suggestions. To do this, we must first examine the child's understanding of death, consider the needs of the family, and caring for the dying child at home. Prenatal and sudden infant death are also mentioned. Finally, the psychological needs of nursing staff involved in caring for dying children are discussed.

CHILDREN'S UNDERSTANDING OF DEATH

Chapter 4 discusses how children learn to understand their world and mature cognitively and the influence of Piaget's theory of cognitive development was emphasized in relationship to children's understanding of illness. A similar approach has been adopted in studying children's perception of death (Goodall, 1994; Rathbone, 1996), although this topic has received only limited investigation. This is not surprising as it is clearly difficult to carry out work of this kind with young children, particularly as it is hard to know if it distresses children to question them about the nature of death.

A number of studies have shown how children's understanding of death is linked to age. Gonda and Ruark (1984) suggest that up until the age of 2 years it is difficult to know whether children are aware of death or its meaning. Between the ages of 2 and 5 years, children seem unable to separate death from fantasy and find it difficult to understand that it happens to everybody, including themselves. At this age they have very little information about death and dying, often seeing it as a reversible process.

Lansdown and Benjamin (1985) in their study of 5–9 year old children, found that 60 per cent of children studied had a complete or almost complete concept of death, and by the age of 8 or 9 years almost all children had a fully developed notion of death. However, although there is some awareness of the causes and finality of death, it is still considered as a remote possibility. It must be remembered that this kind of description is very broad and that many children will show understanding at an earlier or later age than suggested above.

A more precise way of categorizing children's understanding of death is that based upon stages of cognitive development, rather than age alone. Reilly *et al.* (1983) have studied children's understanding of death and personal mortality in relation to cognitive developmental factors. As would be expected, children at more advanced cognitive levels gave more sophisticated answers to questions concerning death and dying. In their research, Reilly *et al.* found that all the children between the ages of 5 and 10 years they investigated, who could conserve, believed in personal mortality (see Chapter 4 for a full discussion of the nature of conservation). However, over half of those children who could not conserve also believed in personal mortality. This study suggests that many young children with a serious illness can understand the idea of their own death. How they conceive of death is often dependent upon their language ability.

Cadranell (1994), in Hill's comprehensive book about dying, notes that pre-school children (at Piaget's pre-operational level of cognitive development) do not have a complete concept of death. Andrewes and Taylor (1995) discuss how they associate death with disappearance, leaving, sleep, or 'going somewhere' (p. 177), although some children as young as 3 or 4 years old may have some concept. This association with leaving or going somewhere is hardly surprising given the adult preoccupation of avoiding words such as death or dying and using metaphors such as 'left us', 'gone', 'passed away' and 'loss/lost'. Likewise, the linking of death with sleep is not difficult to fathom and may reflect words or phrases they have heard adults use ('fell asleep', 'the big sleep'). It does seem though that the child's concept of death does develop according to broad Piagetian principles. However, as Cadranell (1994) points out, other conditions may speed up this developmental process. In particular, personal experience of death is of course likely to affect children's understanding and responses to dying. Cadranell writes (p. 35):

Amongst healthy children the concept of death evolves gradually and there is a wide variety of attitudes and ideas. This process is speeded up when children are exposed to death at an early age.

Those children who experience someone close to them dying have greater knowledge about death and seem to have a more realistic notion of their own death. Clearly children can learn about death, depending to some extent upon their experience and level of cognitive development. This makes it imperative for nurses to collect as much information about children in their care as is possible within the constraints of their job. It must be appreciated that, although there are stages which children pass through, within these stages there is a wide range of individual differences (see Chapter 5). These vary according to the cognitive experiences and emotional life history of each individual child.

DYING CHILDREN'S AWARENESS OF DEATH

The extent to which children who are dying are aware of their impending death is a delicate topic. It is not an area in which a great deal of research has been carried out, and yet at a practical level nurses do have to deal with this situation. This might easily lead to the topic being avoided altogether, and to rather uncomfortable situations between children, nurses and parents. Andrewes and Taylor (1995) describe the 'curtain of silence' in which all the parties involved pretend that everything is normal and that nothing is happening. This is based upon the desire to be protective and to avoid what might appear to be unnecessary distress. The charade may equally involve the dying child who may wish to protect his or her parents from the truth.

However, a study by Bluebond–Langer (1989) of the dying child and siblings' awareness of death, suggests that dying children can often appreciate the seriousness of the illness they are facing. Bluebond–Langer describes fatally ill children as being aware that the illness being faced is no ordinary one, despite the fact that parents and others have not informed them of the severity of their illness. She suggests that these children undergo a process of discovery. Jones (1990) in his work with children with haemophilia who are HIV positive describes similar findings.

If this is the case, there are important implications concerning the way in which nurses and others communicate with the fatally ill child. Any tendency to avoid the issue might lead to an eventual loss of trust. Elsegood (1996) suggests that a guiding principle is to be honest, sensitive and non-judgemental. The wishes of the family should be respected. Elsegood also warns about making assumptions that the child should only be told when they ask – this relies too heavily on adults perceiving cues from the child. Similarly, Cadranell (1994) supports the notion that children need to be given opportunities to discuss what is happening to them even if they do not choose to take those opportunities at a particular time. Cadranell suggests that this does not impose an additional burden on the child but gives permission 'to talk about what is already on their minds' (p. 37).

It is important then to provide the right opportunities for talking in an open manner but without being probing or over-powering. There are a number of personal accounts of how parents cope with the death of a child and, for nurses having to face this situation, they provide much insight into the dying child's needs. Hill (1994), Lindsay and Elsegood (1996) and Katz and Sidell (1994) all give examples of how parents have experienced the death of a child, conveying the feelings of the people involved and indicating the role health professionals might play in this process.

THE NEEDS OF THE FAMILY

Bluebond–Langer (1989) writes:

The victims of chronic and terminal illness are not limited to the diagnosed patient. The destructive effects of such diseases spread to the families of those inflicted.

Cadranell (1994) stresses that the job of the health professional is not only to care for the sick child, but for the family as well. A survey by Lovell (1983) of mothers whose babies had died indicates the lack of support they received from professionals. In particular it was felt that hospital staff discouraged them, inadvisably, from talking about their loss. Similarly, in a personal account of caring for her own dying son at home, Bennett (1984) describes the lack of communication experienced between carers. Her account emphasizes the need of families with dying children for continuity of care. This can best be achieved if families are nursed, as far as possible, by a primary nurse or at least a stable team of nurses each time they are admitted to hospital. Community child care nurses (see Chapter 11) can help to bridge the communication gap and health visitors and other carers should be encouraged to visit and communicate with hospital nurses. Ross-Alaolmolki (1985) stresses the importance of communication between the child who is dying, the family and the caregivers. Continuity of care will undoubtedly facilitate this.

Wilkinson (1994) emphasizes the different ways in which individual family members react to the death of a child. Their reactions are made even more unpredictable as, in many cases, death is sudden and the family are unprepared. Furthermore, it is important to bear in mind that not only the parents will need careful consideration and support, but also all those involved with the family, including grandparents, siblings and friends, and others within the child's community. In particular, there is the danger of other children in the family being neglected, without there being adequate explanation, as stressed by Zyrinsky (1994). A common reaction by parents, which is referred to a great deal, is that of guilt, particularly when death is as the result of a genetic illness (Clarke, 1994). In some ways parents often see themselves as responsible for the death of their child. The real impact of a child's death on the family is brought home by Gonda and Ruark (1984) who point out that the breakup of the family often follows.

Clearly, there are limitations to what nurses can do. Ideally they should be able to become involved in both hospital and home care, as appropriate. The use of outside agencies such as social workers and knowledge of supportive agencies such as Cruse are helpful. Nurses certainly need to get to know the individual problems facing the family and to be supportive in helping to resolve them. These suggestions point to the need for nurses to be given sufficient time and autonomy to help support the family. In nursing the dying child it may be that time is all they have to give, and this kind of involvement needs official recognition. The support required by individual families will clearly differ and 'what works for one family may not work for another' (Cadranell, 1994, p. 39).

To conclude this section on the needs of the family, it is important to

Cruse, National Organization for the Widowed and their Children, Cruse House, 126 Sheen Road, Richmond, Surrey, TW9 1UR. Tel: 0181-940 4818/9047.

emphasize that nurses must not judge family members who do not react to the death of a child, as they would themselves. Sister Frances Dominica (1987) in her informative and very moving paper about her experiences at Helen House, the first children's hospice in England, writes:

> *One relative may remain dry eyed and controlled throughout; the other hysterical and seemingly out of control. We have to accept both and not be thrown off balance by either. To whom is the hysterical reaction of a newly bereaved teenager a threat? In the privacy of a room can that young person not be allowed to lie down beside the dead brother or sister or hold the child or scream to God to bring this person he or she loves back to life again?*

CARING FOR THE DYING CHILD AT HOME

The possibility of home care for the dying child has already been touched upon and the need to foster communication between all the caring agencies involved stressed. Goldman *et al.* (1990) describe the work of the 'symptom care team' at the Hospitals for Sick Children in London, which is involved at all stages with children who have cancer, both in hospital and in the community. It is their view that children almost always prefer to die at home where they can be in familiar surroundings, being cared for by their family. The team, because they are involved with the family from the time of diagnosis, have usually established firm links with them which means that parents do not have to constantly build new relationships when they are faced with the stress of knowing that active treatment has ceased. By providing a 24 hour 'on call' system, the team are available to families if difficulties or concerns arise. The growth of community child care nursing teams (see Chapter 11) also provides families with the support they need to be able to care confidently for a dying child at home, as a realistic option to hospital care. This option may be beneficial, not only to the dying child, but also to the family. Research into the effects of caring for a dying child suggests that the longer term problems experienced by parents and siblings may be reduced if the child is nursed at home (Lauer *et al.*, 1983). However, it must be acknowledged that for some parents having a dying child at home is not something they can cope with either physically or psychologically.

A further way to provide family care for the dying child is the provision of hospice care. In a chapter about the role of the hospice by Hill (1994), she suggests that the hospice can offer support in a flexible way according to individual needs. Support is offered to all members of the family, some who may not have experienced death before. Whilst more parents choose death at home for their child, many prefer that their child should die in the supportive environment of the hospice. Rooms are equipped so that all members of the family (including pets) can be together. One particular advantage of a hospice, as compared to a hospital, is that its function is entirely to devote time to the children and their families. It may also help parents look beyond the death and to maintain an appropriate life style for other family members, especially any siblings.

Deciding where to care for a dying child is a personal matter involving the child, parents and health professionals, and although research can help us make more informed decisions, in the end, it is still an emotional response. But the lack of investigations undertaken to evaluate home and hospital care does make it even more difficult to decide wisely. Death is still a difficult topic to approach and to wish to undertake research in the area might seem to be insensitive. Yet, the more we know the more we can help and, in particular, it will help us to explain to parents whether more of their fears are likely to be true. These often concern whether it is possible practically to care for the dying child at home and the emotional strain it will impose. This in itself might help parents decide for themselves what is best for their child and the family.

PRENATAL DEATH

Capper (1982) in her short and delicate discussion of the loss of a baby notes:

> *A stillbirth leaves its mark on the parents' hearts for life and whether it becomes an open wound or a healed scar greatly depends on the circumstances at the time.*

Up until relatively recent times 'conventional wisdom' suggested that stillbirths should be forgotten about as quickly as possible (Katz and Sidell, 1994). However, the Stillbirth and Neonatal Death Society (SANDS) has raised awareness of the immense trauma of stillbirth and miscarriage which has led to a reappraisal of professional approaches to this delicate area. The care which parents receive around the time of the death can greatly influence the longer term outcomes (e.g. the open wound or healed scar described by Capper above).

It is suggested that a common reaction is a feeling of anger and guilt attributable to the unhappy combination of birth and death together. In a very thoughtful review Hopper (1994) stresses that mourning is more difficult as the family have little if any knowledge of the child as a separate being. She suggests that the needs of the parents should be followed as much as possible after a stillborn child. They may wish to wash and dress the baby, collect mementos such as a lock of hair and have a photograph taken of the baby or of themselves with the baby which can help them remember at some later stage that their baby was a person. Many parents spend time just holding the baby which can be helpful. One bereaved father wrote (White, 1997):

> *We had 15 hours of holding his body, which still held the memory of the beauty of his spirit. Fifteen hours to quench our need for his*

*physical presence, to touch and be touched, and to warm him with
our warmth.*

Some parents may also wish to take their baby home and arrange the
funeral. Whatever course of action parents wish to take Mallinson
(1989) feels that parents should be positively encouraged to say goodbye
to their baby, and the option should be put to parents on more than one
occasion with 'care and sensitivity'. She feels that parents may, at a later
stage, regret not being involved with the final decisions and physical
tasks that need doing. Along with Capper, it is noted by Harrington
(1982) that it might be best to leave the clearing away of the baby things
at home to the parents. As Capper aptly puts it:

> *It is necessary that the baby's death is accepted for the process of
> learning to live again to begin.*

This need to mourn is a common theme in much of the research in this
area. The importance of follow up on discharge from hospital is also
emphasized. Hopper (1994) discusses that parents are not always given
the chance to talk through their loss, and the need for community involvement is stressed. The family (including grandparents and siblings)
should have a named person (e.g. midwife, health visitor) with whom
they can establish a personal relationship and have the opportunity to
discuss their loss. Caring agencies such as the Stillbirth and Neonatal
Death Society or the Foundation for the Study of Infant Deaths, are
helpful and again nursing personnel may initiate this contact. SANDS,
for example, produce an excellent leaflet which parents can send to
friends and family which gives information about how they can support
the bereaved parents. Hopper (1994) also notes the father may find it a
particularly difficult time as he may find that his own grieving is
suppressed because he is expected to cope and be 'strong'.

**Stillbirth and Neonatal Death
Society**, 28 Portland Place,
London WI 4DE. Tel: 0171-436
5881.
**Foundation for the Study of
Infant Deaths** (Cot Death
Research and Support), 35
Belgrave Square, London SWIX
8QB. Tel: 0171-235 1721.

Although not clearly defined, it does seem that the role of the nurse
is crucial in helping parents who have experienced the loss of a baby. To
some extent we have to rely on the personal capabilities and initiative of
the nursing staff. It is not possible to legislate for the reactions of parents
and for the way nurses become involved in this process. Flexibility must
be encouraged and an awareness that the nurse's responsibility is to the
whole family and not just to the parents in one specific clinical setting,
that is the hospital.

SUDDEN INFANT DEATH

Sudden infant deaths or 'cot deaths' raise similar problems for the
parents as does the stillborn child. The trauma experienced by these
parents is particularly acute as the lack of cause can lead to confusion
and 'irrational guilt' (Hindmarch, 1994). As Limerick (1982) points out,
unlike stillbirths, the vast majority of cot deaths occur at home and this
she notes is likely to make the parents feel wholly responsible. She

suggests that the effects are likely to be more severe and long lasting and that this is partly the result of the feeling that they might have prevented the death.

In a more detailed review of the impact of sudden infant death on the family, Nikolaisen (1981), an American assistant professor of nursing, discusses the specific role of the nurse. She describes in detail the predictable reactions of the parents, which include feelings of guilt and emotional responses. These emotional responses are often reflected in depressive behaviour, which Nikolaisen suggests should not be interpreted as undesirable. The longer term effects on the family are discussed. She reports research which shows that mothers often experience wide mood swings and may find interpersonal relationships more difficult. Similarly, some research suggests that fathers may immerse themselves in work to avoid contact at home with their partners. It is also important, she notes, to help parents recognize the needs of others in their family, especially siblings, and to avoid getting too caught up in their own grief.

The implications for nursing care are considerable. As Nikolaisen argues, 'nurses are especially qualified to counsel grieving families'. She reports a study carried out in the USA which involved nurses interviewing parents who had experienced a cot death. It was found that the nurse who conducted the interviews was providing not only information to parents, but counselling as well. On the basis of this, a systematic programme to provide support has been set up with the aim of offering preventive mental health care. It has been found that the nurse can help in explaining the cause of death as much as possible and in allowing parents to talk through their experiences. To some extent they also help to normalize the grief process by pointing out how others have dealt with similar situations. The positive effects of their form of intervention have led to legislation being passed for each state, territory, and possession, to have a similar programme involving the community nurse. Maybe a similar approach will have to be adopted to provide this kind of service in the UK. Although it is not possible to legislate for the process of mourning, it is possible to ensure that all families are offered long term professional support.

Health visitors also have a major role with parents who have subsequent babies following sudden infant death. The *Care of the Next Infant (CONI)* programme is now widely established in the UK. The CONI programme aims to provide organized support for families who have suffered a previous sudden infant death. Parents are interviewed during the antenatal period and are informed about the programme. Parents are offered a range of support including weekly visits from the health visitor, apnoea monitor, room thermometer, scales and a symptom diary (Waite, 1994; Baumer and McLindon, 1994). The programme is well received by parents who gain vital emotional support as well as practical help. On a positive note, sudden infant death has been the focus of an enormous amount of research that has led to recommendations being made which have reduced the incidence of sudden infant death significantly over the last decade. Of particular interest is the *Confidential Enquiry into Stillbirths and Deaths in Infancy (CESDI)* (1996) which has reported annually since 1994. Research has focussed on sudden infant death in three regions in England and comprises case controls (whereby each child who dies is matched with three healthy controls), an expert panel (who identify any contributing factors) and an autopsy enquiry. Each year the Confidential Enquiry has published recommendations for parents and health professionals after analysis of the data. Such recommendations have included advice about the sleeping positions of babies, temperature, exposure to cigarette smoke and head covering. This type of large scale research which is a collaborative venture by a consortium of professional groups is an excellent example of research which has made a real and significant difference to practice.

COPING WITH DEATH

Brewis (1990) in her discussion of the terminal care of children with cancer makes some practical suggestions which nurses may find useful. One very sensible suggestion made by this author is that members of the team who are not on duty at the time of the child's death are warned prior to returning to the ward so that they are not 'caught unawares'. There are few more distressing experiences than meeting the parents of a child when you are not aware that the child has recently died. Brewis stresses how important it is that nurses cope with the death of a child in a way that is appropriate at the time. On p. 165, she emphasizes that:

> ... *what is said and how one behaves are important to the parents, as they will remember this time for the rest of their lives.*

However, none of us know how we will feel when faced with a child's death, nor can we say with confidence that we have the ability to offer the support needed by the family, as well as coping with the other children and families on a ward.

The final consideration in coping with death is to recognize that those closely involved with the care of the dying child and who provide support for the family, also have needs of their own. Capewell (1996) stresses the importance of planning an organizational response to reduce stress and provide support for staff. She suggests that such a response involves preparation prior to the death of the child and involves, among other things, self-awareness. Capewell and Beattie (1996) discuss further ways in which professionals can help care for themselves and other staff through a range of strategies. Clearly education is key in this process and there are a number of post-registration programmes available to help practitioners to understand their own responses better, and the responses of others, to the death of a child.

- It is imperative to avoid deceit when working with the dying child and the family. The moment untruths are allowed to slip in to the relationship, it is predictable that a lack of trust will emerge and the delicate relationship will be put in jeopardy.
- It is important to be guided by the child and the parents and to maintain a relationship within the guidelines they provide. Nurses will have their own values, but should try to avoid imposing them onto the situation as far as possible.
- Professional care should be extended to the whole family. This should be continuous and be maintained in the community until the needs of those involved have been resolved to their satisfaction. This may well need to be a policy consideration of the whole paediatric unit. Individual nurses may be unable to initiate such a programme alone.
- Nurses involved with the dying child must recognize their own and each other's emotional needs and take positive steps to ensure that these are being met. A continuing programme of death education for those involved is extremely important in helping nurses manage their professional role.
- The practical requirements of nurses involved with dying children must be recognized and time given to ensure that they can be carried out. One example might be weekly meetings. This is likely to involve giving both considerable autonomy and flexibility to the nursing staff. One cannot expect sensitive and intelligent care for the dying if nurses are not given full responsibility for their actions.

REFERENCES

Andrewes, C. and Taylor, D. (1995) Death and Dying: a healthy response, in *Adolescence: Caring for Health*, (ed. A. Fatchett), Baillière Tindall, London.

Baumer, D. and McLindon, H. (1994) Support after cot death: the CONI programme in action. *Professional Care of Mother and Child*, 4(5), 131–3.

Bennett, P. (1984) A care team for terminally ill children. *Nursing Times*, 80(10), 26–7.

Bluebond–Langer, M. (1989) Worlds of dying children and their well siblings. *Death Studies*, 13 1–16.

Brewis, E.L. (1990) Care of the terminally ill child, *The Child with Cancer*, (ed. J. Thompson), Scutari Press, London.

Cadranell, J. (1994) Talking about Death – Parents and Children, in *Caring for Dying Children and their Families*, (ed. L. Hill), Chapman and Hall, London.

Capewell, E. (1996) Planning and Organisational Response, in *Working with Children in Grief*, (eds B. Lindsay and J. Elsegood), Baillière Tindall, London.

Capewell, E. and Beattie, L. (1996) Staff Care and Support, in *Working with Children in Grief*, (eds B. Lindsay and J. Elsegood), Baillière Tindall, London.

Capper, E. (1982) Stillbirth. *Nursing* Series, 1(34), 1490.

CESDI (Confidential Enquiries into Stillbirths and Deaths in Infancy) (1996) 3rd Annual Report. *Maternal and Childhealth Research Consortium*, London.

Clarke, A. (1994) Dying from Genetic Disease, in *Caring for Dying Children and their Families*, (ed. L. Hill), Chapman and Hall, London.

Dominica, Sister Frances (1987) Reflections on death in childhood. *British Medical Journal*, **294**, 108–10.

Elsegood, J. (1996) Breaking Bad News to Children, in *Working with Children in Grief and Loss*, (eds B. Lindsay and J. Elsegood), Baillière Tindall, London.

Goldman, A., Beardsmore, S. and Hunt, J. (1990) Palliative care for children with cancer – home, hospital, or hospice. *Archives of Disease in Childhood*, **65**, 641–3.

Gonda, T.A. and Ruark, J.E. (1984) *Dying Dignified. The Health Professional's Guide to Care*, Addison-Wesley, Menlo Park, CA.

Goodall, J. (1994) Thinking like a child about death and dying, in *Caring for Dying Children and their Families*, (ed. L. Hill), Chapman and Hall, London.

Harrington, V. (1982) Bereavement and childbirth: Look, listen and support. *Nursing Mirror*, **154**(2), 21–8.

Hill, L. (ed.) (1994) *Caring for Dying Children and their Families*, Chapman and Hall, London.

Hindmarch, C. (1994) Sudden Death, in *Caring for Dying Children and their Families*, (ed. L. Hill), Chapman and Hall, London.

Hopper, E. (1994) Perinatal Death, in *Caring for Dying Children and their Families*, (ed. L. Hill), Chapman and Hall, London.

Jones, P. (1990) *Living with Haemophilia*, 3rd edn, Castle House Publications, Tunbridge Wells.

Katz, J. and Sidell, M. (1994) *Easeful Death: Caring for Dying and Bereaved People*, Hodder and Stoughton, London.

Lansdown, R. and Benjamin, G. (1985) The development of the concept of death in children aged 5–9 years. *Childcare and Development*, **11**, 13–20.

Lauer, M.E., Mulhern, R.K., Wallskog, J.M. and Carnitta, B.M. (1983) A comparison study of parental adaptation following a child's death at home or in the hospital. *Pediatrics*, **71**(1), 107–12.

Limerick, S. (1982) Cot deaths. *Nursing* Series, **1**(34), 1491–3.

Lindsay, B. and Elsegood, J. (1996) *Working with Children in Grief and Loss* Baillière Tindall, London.

Lovell, A. (1983) A bereavement with a difference: a study of late miscarriage, stillbirth and prenatal death, *South Bank, Sociology Occasional Paper 4*, Social Sciences Department, Polytechnic of the South Bank, London.

Mallinson, G. (1989) When a baby dies. *Nursing Times* **85**(93), 1–4.

Nikolaisen, S. (1981) The impact of sudden infant death on the family: Nursing intervention. *Topics in Clinical Nursing*, **3**(3), 45–53.

Rathbone, B. (1996) Developmental Perspectives, in *Working with Children in Grief*, (eds B. Lindsay and J. Elsegood), Baillière Tindall, London.

Reilly, T.P., Hasazi, J.E. and Bond, L.A. (1983) Children's conceptions of death and personal mortality. *Journal of Pediatric Psychology*, **8**, 21–31.

Ross-Alaolmolki, K. (1985) Supportive care for families of dying children. *The Nursing Clinics of North America*, **20**(2), 457–67.

Waite, A.J. (1994) After a cot death: the impact of CONI. *Professional Care of Mother and Child*, **4**(5), 127–8.

White, M. (1997) Personal Communication.

Wilkinson, T. (1994) The Extended Family and other carers, in *Caring for Dying Children and their Families*, (ed. L. Hill), Chapman and Hall, London.

Zyrinsky, L. (1994) Brothers and Sisters, in *Caring for Dying Children and their Families*, (ed. L. Hill), Chapman and Hall, London.

The following three texts provide excellent reviews of work undertaken in this field. The works of Hill and Lindsay/Elsegood are written specifically in relation to children whereas Katz and Sidell's book is more general.

Hill, L. (ed.) (1994) *Caring for Dying Children and their Families*, Chapman and Hall, London.

Katz, J. and Sidell, M. (1994) *Easeful Death: Caring for Dying and Bereaved People*, Hodder and Stoughton, London.

Lindsay, B. and Elsegood, J. (eds) (1996) *Working with Children in Grief and Loss*, Baillière Tindall, London.

16 RESEARCH INTO PRACTICE: FINAL CONSIDERATIONS

This book has brought together a great deal of research from the fields of psychology and nursing, which is of particular relevance to those health professionals charged with the care of children. The main thrust of our argument is that the management of a sick child demands a wide range of specialized skills and knowledge, including the practical use of psychology. Caring for another person is not purely a physical or a medical matter, but one which demands an understanding of the evolving relationships between two or more people. In this sense we believe that proper care cannot be given to children in medical settings unless health professionals understand the psychological aspects of their work. Further, we believe that it is essential that this knowledge be translated into the provision of practical support, that is turning research into practice.

In each chapter we have specified the main practical implications resulting from our discussion. We have done this to emphasize that psychology is a practical discipline and one which can offer guidelines on how to act in specific situations. Sometimes psychologists have not been assertive enough in providing such information and some readers may feel that we have gone too far and been prescriptive in our advice. To some extent this was deliberate in that, if we could not have offered practical advice, the book would not have been worth writing, let alone reading. We are convinced that the suggestions we have made are of value and that they have been based on a body of knowledge derived from research.

It has also become clear to us in writing this book that a number of broader *themes* were recurring in each chapter. Although not as specific as the practical implications drawn out at the end of each chapter, they did appear to be useful as broad guidelines for helping turn theory into practice. In all, seven clear themes emerged, although inevitably some overlap between them was apparent. The themes were as follows: influences on the development of children; how children understand their world; the need to treat each child as an individual; the role of the family; the effects of a child's illness on others; the need to integrate physical and psychological care; and the importance of research findings. We feel that these themes are of sufficient importance to warrant further discussion. The aim of this final chapter is to do just that with the view to pulling together the diverse topics discussed in the previous chapters.

INFLUENCES ON THE DEVELOPING CHILD

In a number of chapters the wide range of influences on the developing child have been brought to the reader's attention. Special consideration has been given to very early experiences and in particular to the young child's initial interactions with caregivers. The role of other people in helping to socialize the very young child stands out clearly, as does the young child's need for a variety of stimulating experiences. Although it is stating the obvious to point out that these influences are multifactorial, that is derived from an unspecifiable variety of sources, it remains nonetheless an important point.

Take for example the continuing debate about the effects of separation on young children. The research shows clearly that there is more than just one factor that needs consideration. First, separation itself needs careful analysis. Do we mean short term, medium term or long term separation? Is it permanent or temporary? Is this a new experience or is the child used to being parted from known and trusted people? Having answered questions of this nature, the researcher must then focus on a wide range of other factors. It is clearly crucial that some assessment should be made of the quality of the relationship the child has with home. A child from a supportive background may find short term separation a valuable experience as indeed may a child from a nonsupportive home. The child's own personality (including ways of coping) is of course another factor. Perhaps more importantly an attempt must be made to consider separation from the child's perspective, as this view is more likely to determine behaviour. Therefore, in researching this important question, a whole range of factors must be taken into consideration and a simple analysis of the effects of separation is not easy to undertake. This brings us back to the point that any relationship between a child's experiences and subsequent behaviour must be seen as multifactorial. Hence, health professionals need to be careful (as must psychologists) in stating simple one-to-one relationships between apparently discrete factors, for example a child's behaviour and separation.

What this means in practice is that the environment is critically important in children's development. It is crucial that great care be taken in creating physical and psychological environments for children. This is particularly true for those children in a strange, potentially traumatic situation such as hospital. Nursing personnel need to give much thought and imagination to producing creative environments which have the potential to enhance children's development. This is not to be taken lightly, as a major point emerging from our discussion is the importance of experience on development. Hence, any situation the child faces is one in which we must practise our psychological knowledge. It is the responsibility of health professionals caring for children to minimize any traumatic effects and to enhance the learning experiences of any child through manipulating the environment.

A CHILD'S EYE VIEW

Children perceive and understand their world in different ways from adults. It is in fact quite difficult for adults to see the world the same way as children do and it has taken a whole range of intricate experiments by people such as Piaget to help us appreciate some of the differences. What is clear is that children do impose their own order on the world and do not experience it as a random collection of happenings. It is important that we appreciate children's own viewpoints even if we cannot necessarily share them. The way they deal with the world is not inferior, only different.

Linked to this is the finding that age alone is not the only determinant of a child's level of understanding. Children progress through certain stages of cognitive growth which are not tightly tied to age. There is a danger in assuming that all 3 year old children are alike, whereas in fact at that age there will be a whole range of differing skills and abilities displayed. Age is an obvious and easy means of trying to find out about a child and is often a good and readily available starting point. However, it is necessary to be very sensitive to individual differences, as illustrated in Part One of this book and in particular in Chapter 5.

The key point is that children are *active* in making sense of their environment. They do not simply respond in a passive sense, but create their own understanding and participate in a constructive way. In this sense any experience is subject to the way in which individual children interpret it. It is difficult to generalize and to talk about a group of children responding in a similar way to a given situation. From your own experience you will know how children see things differently. For example, you only have to ask them to talk about a set of drawings to appreciate the richness of imagination individual children express. It is this individual uniqueness that is important in appreciating a child's eye view of the world.

This uniqueness is particularly evident in how children respond to the whole array of events associated with hospitalization. Chapter 4 provides an interesting example of how certain words such as 'organ' or 'tissue' can be misinterpreted from a nonmedical perspective. How children respond to hospitalization may, to some extent, be a function of how they construct say the ward situation. The more 'fun-like' it is, the more likely it is that they might interpret it in a positive way. As emphasized in Part Two, it is the fact that hospitals are viewed differently which contributes to the discontinuity between home and hospital. A particularly sensitive issue is children's understanding of death, and we have quoted a number of examples showing how individual children impose their own meanings on the world. Some of these very moving accounts provide clear examples of the uniqueness of children's understanding of this event. In the same way, separation can be seen as a positive, negative or a neutral experience, depending on the meaning children attach to it. These examples help illustrate the need to repeat the individual child's viewpoint in adjusting to any new situation and further emphasize how important it is that health professionals are aware of these factors.

THE INDIVIDUAL APPROACH

Although this is very obvious, we do feel it is worth stressing separately. The two themes already discussed, influences on the development of children and how children understand their world, lead clearly to the conclusion that each child is unique and requires individual care. This means that the needs of each child have to be carefully identified and, where possible, provision made to meet them. In this sense we are talking about making individual care plans in which to try and incorporate the total experiences of the child. This is in essence what the nursing process is concerned with and we find ourselves lending support to this approach from a research as well as a practical perspective. It seems to us that when cared for by other people, children – like adults – have the right to expect an approach which focusses on their psychological as well as their physical needs. This requires a totally individual approach, despite the conflicting demands of other more routine nursing tasks. It seems to us important that any conflict between the provision of individual care and hospital efficiency is resolved in favour of the former, in this case the child patient. Although we have presented this theme only briefly, it is not our intention to play it down. In our view it is of major importance despite the administrative burden it may impose.

THE ROLE OF THE FAMILY

In many of the chapters in this book, considerable emphasis is placed on the role the family can play when nursing children. We feel very strongly that, despite continuous pleas to see parents as equal partners, not enough as yet has been achieved. This gives grounds for considerable concern and, throughout the book, we have shown the range of skills possessed by parents in caring for their children. Parents appreciate more than anybody the uniqueness of their own children and perhaps more importantly have evolved strategies for dealing with them as individuals. From the other side of the fence, the child too will have learned how to cope with and respond to a unique set of parenting skills. It seems to us important that this negotiated understanding be incorporated into the nursing situation in order to optimize the child's physical and psychological welfare.

On the other hand, we recognize that this view does present some difficulties for hospital administration. If nurses are to spend more time providing emotional support to those children whose parents are not there, and in supporting the parents who are, more staffing is likely to be required. At the same time, it is not easy to accept a position which suggests that many parents may be better at caring psychologically for their children, as well as being as good at caring for them physically, with advice. The point here is that, through skilful cooperation with parents and other family members, the job of the nurse can actually be made easier, providing sufficient resources are made available to implement such a policy. It is always important to remember that, for most children, parents have to take over the nursing role very quickly when they are discharged from hospital. Our suggestion goes some way towards helping integrate hospital with home care.

A particular issue which has caused considerable concern in the past is of course visiting children when they are in hospital. This is briefly discussed in Chapter 1 and referred to extensively in Part Two. In previous editions of this book we focussed on restrictions to visiting as being wholly detrimental to the wellbeing of the sick child. There is no need to have any restrictions at all on visiting children and on spending time with them and since the first edition of this book in 1986 we have seen major changes which are wholeheartedly welcomed. Hospitals, after all, not only serve the community but are in fact owned by its members. It has, at last, become evident that any approach to restricting the legitimate access of parents is an inhibiting factor in the recovery process for children.

EFFECTS OF A CHILD'S ILLNESS ON OTHERS

At the same time as appearing to advocate a withdrawal from the traditional nursing role, by allowing parents more involvement, we also wish to suggest an area in which the role of nurses is being extended. It is clear that in many cases having an ill child in the family affects other people. These include parents, siblings, other family members, the child's friends and sometimes of course the nursing staff. There is no doubt that ill children do make considerable physical and mental demands on their parents. Many parents find themselves, for example, travelling long distances to visit the hospital, having to keep a home going, looking after other family members, while at the same time trying to provide proper care for their sick child. In this sense then, parents themselves may be in need of some support or constructive help which might be best recognized and provided by nursing staff. Although this imposes yet another strain on nurses they are in a very good position to help and, in so doing, can indirectly benefit the child patient.

Others too can be affected by a child's illness. There may be the danger that the problems of the ill child take over to the extent that the needs of siblings are overlooked and, perhaps by involving them in the routine care of their ill brother or sister, this might be avoided. Certainly every effort has to be made to ensure that siblings do not in any way feel themselves being deprived and nurses can help by bringing this to the attention of parents. Clearly, there has to be some limit on the responsibility of the nurse in situations such as this. However, it is likely to be of considerable help to the patient if the effects on others can be minimized.

It is also important to bear in mind the effects on nurses themselves. We suspect it is particularly stressful nursing children because of the kind of care required and the somewhat emotional responses young children evoke in us, especially when they are ill. This issue is raised specifically in Chapter 15 on the dying child where the need to provide support for the nursing staff is discussed. It may well be that there is a similar need in other areas of children's nursing and it is important that the needs of nurses are not neglected.

INTEGRATING PHYSICAL AND PSYCHOLOGICAL CARE

Another major theme of the book is the relationship between physical and psychological care. It is our view that the two are complementary and that nurses need to consider both aspects when working with children. We are not suggesting in any way that psychological care should replace physical care. Clearly, in many situations, the physical needs of the child are uppermost and priority must be given to the provision of appropriate medical treatment. However, we hope that this book will show that, in a wide range of nursing situations, psychological considerations are extremely important and, in many cases, influence the responses to physical forms of treatment.

Part One of the book illustrates, for instance, how understanding a child's development can lead to better nursing care. Additionally, a great deal of the material in Part Two on nursing the child and adolescent in hospital and in the community has been derived from nursing research with a strong psychological bias. Even the specific issues discussed in the final part rely on psychological research in order that informed advice can be given. In other words, we think that when considering illness, a purely medical or physical approach is inadequate. In order to make practical implications for nursing clear, we have drawn upon a large body of psychological knowledge. It must always be remembered that the provision of nursing care involves at least one person (the nurse) interacting with another (the patient). This is a psychological not a physical situation and, as such, requires an understanding which is broader than that given by the medical model. Hopefully, this book will provide you, the reader, with sufficient additional knowledge to make a difference to your approach when nursing children.

THE IMPORTANCE OF RESEARCH-BASED KNOWLEDGE VERSUS BELIEFS AND ASSUMPTIONS

We have emphasized throughout the book that psychologists deal with *evidence*. Before trying to come to any decision, to form an opinion, or to give practical advice, psychologists are always seeking to collect data relating to the issue in hand. This can be done using a variety of techniques, ranging from experimentation to interviewing. Because psychology places so much importance on data, it is classified as an *empirical* discipline. Empirical disciplines can be seen as objective rather than subjective, in that there are always some data on which to base any decision. Although the same data might be interpreted slightly differently, they are always available for re-analysis or to be used by others who wish to question the findings. In other words, psychologists have a clear framework within which to apply their knowledge and tend to distrust non-empirical decision-making.

The importance of the way one deals with the world cannot be emphasized too strongly when related to nursing children. In answering all kinds of questions such as 'Can pre-school children understand the concept of death?', 'Are adolescents emotionally affected by hospitalization?', 'In what ways do children react differently to illness?', psychologists set about it systematically with a view to collecting empirical information. They do not base their decisions on custom and practice or 'historical reasons', or on what is viewed by medical personnel as being most convenient. Instead they question any decision in a constructive way by seeking the empirical source for arriving at any verdict. They strive to establish whether or not there is good evidence for implementing a particular practice. If there is no evidence, psychologists are inclined, almost obliged, to challenge the decision and to question the basis for carrying on this way.

There are numerous examples throughout the book where psychological studies have illuminated nursing practice. In Part Two, for example, there is a wealth of data from a wide range of studies, including those undertaken by one of the authors of this book. Many of these findings have been turned into clear recommendations and have been advocated by important pressure groups such as Action for Sick Children (formerly NAWCH). What remains significant is that in many cases the research which has been conducted has been ignored or deliberately rejected. Many health care structures still fail to satisfy the basic needs of children and their families, as Action for Sick Children continue to point out. This seems odd, especially when there is so much pressure on researchers to make their findings useful and of practical value. Is there any obvious reason for this failure of practitioners to implement the findings of research?

As far as we know there are no empirical data on this precise issue, yet all of us in our different fields have come across what we can only call the 'disbelief' phenomenon. For example, however clearly one demonstrates that physical and psychological care are related, especially when dealing with children, the view that physical care must take preference is in so many cases held very forcefully. Often it is true that the view is held for what appear to be extremely good reasons, lack of staff, lack of time, a disinterested nurse manager, a consultant who fails to listen and so forth. But what must be pointed out is that to hold such a view is illogical and cannot be considered rational. If physical care cannot be divorced from psychological welfare, any set of nursing procedures which are implemented must take into account both physical and psychological factors. Logically they cannot be divorced.

One of the aims in writing this book was to encourage health professionals working with children to take seriously the empirical findings relevant to their work. Psychologists have contributed much to our current understanding of children and how to care for them, but, as we demonstrate, there is no need for all decisions to be based purely on beliefs and assumptions. Indeed, there is, in a large number of instances, research-based knowledge relating to the issue in question. We want to emphasize the need for health professionals to behave logically and rationally in taking this information into account in their everyday work with children. In the long term, this can only lead to greater satisfaction not just on the part of consumers (children and their families) but on the part of nursing staff too.

APPENDIX

BOOKS FOR CHILDREN ABOUT HOSPITAL

This book list is prepared by Action for Sick Children. Books are available from booksellers or public libraries.

Topsy and Tim go to Hospital — Jean and Gareth Anderson, Blackie (1988)

Tim bumps his head and has to stay in hospital but he has such a good time there that when Topsy visits him she wants to stay too!

This lively and informative story will reassure young children facing a stay in hospital. This updated version covers the children's feelings very well and acknowledges the value of play.

Spot's Hospital visit — Eric Hill, Heinemann (1987)

Spot and the gang go to visit their friend Steve in hospital, and have fun when Tom disappears and Spot, Helen and Steve set out to find him.

A good book for younger children, with simple language and bold pictures.

Teddy Goes to Theatre — Jane Donnelly, Countryvise Ltd (1992)

This book follows Teddy through hospital and pre-surgical procedures. It is easy to read with clear photographs showing what is happening to Teddy and the medical equipment used.

Suitable for children under seven who are going to have surgery of any kind. Also available to hire on video from Action for Sick Children (£5 for 3 weeks).

Your heart operation — Pamela Barnes and Janet Rathburn, Children's Heart Foundation

This book is easy to read and follows children through the steps involved when they are in hospital for a heart operation. Photographs show equipment used and the clear descriptions of what will happen, and it will help children overcome the fear of such an operation. Also features space to write about their operation and stick a photograph. Suitable for children under 10 years.

Going to casualty — Anne and Harlow Rockwell, Hamish Hamilton (1987)

A little boy sprains his ankle and is taken to casualty.

This book is suitable for introducing children to hospitals in general, with easy to read language for young children, and clear, detailed pictures of equipment used in hospital.

A visit to hospital — Gillian Mercer and Peter Dennis, Kingfisher (1992)

This book follows Amy's short stay for a simple operation. It shows how a hospital is organized and reveals the special jobs done by the people who work there, as they help the patients get well again.

Contains detailed pictures of the hospital and its layout and introduces children to language used in hospital as well as routines and equipment.

At the hospital — Gerald Hawksley, Orchard Books (1993)

A little book which follows the day of a children's ward where Nicky the Bear works.

Easy to read for children aged seven and under.

Going for an X-ray — Dr Anna Thornton (copies available from Action for Sick Children)

This excellent book explains a number of procedures often performed upon children (including x-rays, ultrasound, CT scans). These test are explained in easy language, given easy to understand names, e.g. radio isotopes or 'magic potion' test, has attractive illustrations as well as a 'parent points' section for each procedure. For parents and children to read together.

Harry goes to hospital — Derek Radford, Walker Books (1992) (for J. Sainsbury)

Harry the Hippo has a stomachache and goes to the doctor's then hospital for an operation. This book also shows other features of the Hippo hospital covering children's and babies' wards.

Detailed pictures of the hospital layout and explanations of jobs done by the staff. Suitable for younger children.

Superted and Spottyman in the case of the missing spots — Mike Young (1988). Available from local hospitals & AWCH Wales

Spottyman wakes up to find his spots are disappearing and Superted takes him to hospital to see what is the matter. Could this be the work of arch-enemy Texas Pete?

A book for confident readers or for parents to read to younger children. Contains colouring-in pages, activities and puzzles.

Arnold goes for a DMSA scan

Arnold has an ultrasound
Why Annie needs a blood test
Darren has a very important test (micturating cystourethrogram) all by Jacqueline Collier and Dot MacKinlay, PALS, c/o Paediatric Renal Unit, City Hospital, Nottingham, NG5 1PB

A very useful set of books describing procedures and feelings of children having the particular tests. Good for older children to read, or for parents to read to younger children.

Josie Smith in hospital – Magdalen Nabb, Harper Collins (1993)

Josie goes into hospital to have her tonsils out. So does her friend Eileen, who makes a terrible fuss. But Josie has her panda, Percy, for company and is very brave.

This book is good for newly confident readers who enjoy reading stories by themselves.

In hospital – Daphne Butler, Simon and Schuster Young Books (1990)

A short book for very young children with clear photographs of all aspects of hospital including the doctors and nurses. A good book for preparing a child before a hospital visit, as questions are asked throughout about the reader's feelings and ideas about hospitals, so any problems or fears may be dealt with.

The hospital highway code — Diana Kimpton and Action for Sick Children, Pan Macmillan (1994)

An excellent book for children of all ages, covering all aspects of going into hospital, including what to pack beforehand, a section for teenagers, overcoming embarrassment, how to deal with pain, taking medicine, equipment used, games, limericks, quizzes and more.

Easy to read with funny and informative illustrations.

Children's ward — Helen White, BBC Books (1990)

Follows the experiences of a group of teenagers in a children's ward together.

Taken from the popular children's TV programme, this is a realistic portrayal of life on a children's ward. Suitable for younger teenagers.

Coming round — Anthony Lishak, A & C Black (1989)

An original mix of narrative and poems following the experiences of a boy in hospital after a road accident.

A good book for children of all ages.

Little tree — A story for children with serious medical problems — Joyce C. Mills, Magination Press (1992)

The story tells of a little tree that is damaged in a storm in which two of her branches are broken. The tree is sad to begin with because she has lost her branches but two wizards teach her that she is still beautiful and just looks different, but still has deep roots and a good heart.

This book was written by a therapist who specializes in telling stories as a healing process for children. This book may help to ease younger children's feelings of fear and anxiousness after a serious operation or accident, especially if they are scarred or look different afterwards.

Page references in *italics* indicate illustrations, figures or tables